Healthy Living for a Lifetime

7 Simple Steps to Better Health

Publisher's Note

This book is intended for general information only. It does not constitute medical, legal, or financial advice or practice. The editors of FC&A have taken careful measures to ensure the accuracy and usefulness of the information in this book. While every attempt has been made to assure accuracy, errors may occur. Some websites, addresses, and telephone numbers may have changed since printing. We cannot guarantee the safety or effectiveness of any advice or treatments mentioned. Readers are urged to consult with their professional financial advisors, lawyers, and health care professionals before making any changes.

Any health information in this book is for information only and is not intended to be a medical guide for self-treatment. It does not constitute medical advice and should not be construed as such or used in place of your doctor's medical advice. Readers are urged to consult with their health care professionals before undertaking therapies suggested by the information in this book, keeping in mind that errors in the text may occur as in all publications and that new findings may supersede older information.

The publisher and editors disclaim all liability (including any injuries, damages, or losses) resulting from the use of the information in this book.

Trust in the Lord with all your heart
and lean not on your own understanding;
in all your ways submit to him,
and he will make your paths straight.

Proverbs 3:5

FC&A Medical Publishing®
103 Clover Green
Peachtree City, GA 30269

Produced by the staff of FC&A
ISBN 978-1-935574-36-1

Table of Contents

Step 1: Choose to be well

Step 2: Eat to heal

Step 3: Lose the fat

Step 1: Choose to be well

Mind your health

What is with you no matter where you go, what you eat, or what your job is? What is not in a pill, or found in a hospital or doctor's office, but is more powerful than you can possibly imagine, impacting your health in hundreds of ways?

It's your attitude. Your feelings and beliefs. Your will. Experts believe these are the vital links between mental and physical health. In other words, the part of you that is made up of emotional, social, spiritual, and behavioral factors plays a major role in how healthy or sick you are.

Let's start with a small, common example. Say you are watching a scary movie. As the tension mounts, you feel a prickling along your scalp. Your palms get a little sweaty. Your heart starts to race. You haven't consciously done anything, but when your brain receives thoughts of fear — the emotion — it tells your body to go on high alert. Your autonomic nervous system (ANS) kicks in. This group of nerves regulates many of the processes you never think about. In this case, it triggers several involuntary responses at once — increased heart rate, sweating, rising blood pressure, and more. Your emotions have just influenced your physical well-being.

While fear like this isn't a disease, it does create stress. And stress can cause or aggravate dozens of conditions, from asthma to cancer.

Here's another example that goes beyond an everyday reaction like fear. A woman in Scotland, recently widowed, experienced what all believed to be a heart attack. Her symptoms included chest pain, shortness of breath, abnormalities in part of her heart, as well as an irregular electrocardiogram. It later turned out this wasn't a heart attack at all, but a well-documented phenomenon called broken heart syndrome — grief so intense it causes a surge of stress hormones to temporarily alter the workings of your heart.

The idea that your emotions can make you sick is not new. More than 15 years ago, the flagship journal of the American Heart Association, *Circulation*, reported "clear and convincing evidence" that certain factors contributed significantly to coronary artery disease (CAD). What were these factors? Depression, anxiety, character traits, social isolation, and chronic stress. In fact, people with heart disease tripled their risk of dying from any cause if they also suffered from anxiety and depression, according to a study in the *Journal of the American Heart Association.*

Now for the good news. If your attitude, feelings, thoughts, beliefs, and emotions can make you sick, they can also make you well. Relaxation with deep breathing, for instance, can lower your blood pressure. Mood-lifting music can lessen headache pain. Humor therapy is commonly used at cancer treatment centers. And reducing stress in general is so beneficial, you could almost call it a cure-all.

A specific collection of therapies designed to make life worth living by increasing personal strengths, boosting positive emotions, and making people feel generally more satisfied in life is called positive psychology. This real branch of science has doctors intrigued. When women with breast cancer participated in positive psychology, many felt they also had more energy and were better able to cope with cancer treatments.

Ancient healing practices always involved the spirit, the mind, AND the body. In fact, the connection between mental and physical health dates as far back as Hippocrates, the Father of Medicine, who wrote, "The natural healing force within each one of us is the greatest force in getting well."

It was only when man discovered bacteria that the world of medicine changed forever. Once early pathologists like Bassi and Pasteur connected microorganisms to disease, the wheels of science rolled over mind-body therapies, crushing them in the wake of vaccines and antibiotics. Medicine became all about the next pill or the next injection.

Many believe we've gone too far in that direction, forgetting the simpler healing powers. But the pendulum may be swinging back. The past 20 years have seen a flood of research exploring how psychological factors play a role in illness, and how mind-body techniques can bring better sleep, lessen stress, boost mood, ease symptoms of disease, and generally improve quality of life.

The bottom line is you are responsible for your own health and well-being in ways that go beyond simple diet and lifestyle choices. Embrace the idea there is a dramatic and powerful connection between your mind and your body, and you can start changing the way you feel.

PARASYMPATHETIC NERVOUS SYSTEM	SYMPATHETIC NERVOUS SYSTEM
Rest & Digest	*Fight or Flight*
Pupils constrict	Pupils dilate
More saliva is produced to help with digestion	Less saliva is produced, so your mouth goes dry
Respiration becomes slow & steady	Breathing becomes fast & shallow
Heart rate slows	Heart beats faster
Blood pressure lowers	Blood pressure rises
Blood vessels dilate	Stomach & intestines slow
Digestion is stimulated	More blood sugar is produced to power muscles
	Adrenalin is released

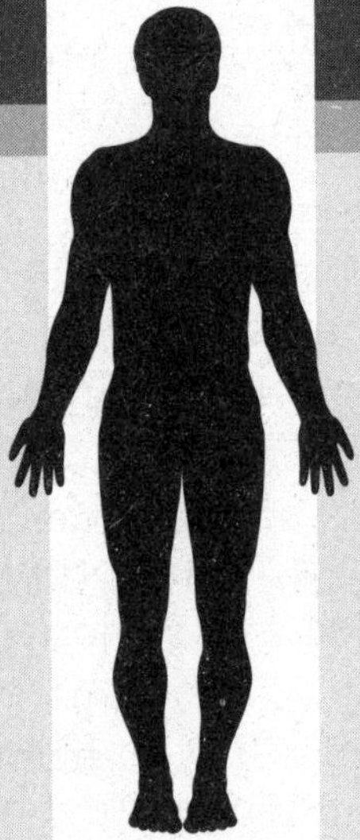

Your autonomic nervous system is made up of two parts, the parasympathetic and sympathetic nervous systems, which respond in completely opposite ways, depending on the situation. This is a great example of how emotions influence your body and can impact your health.

Think well, be well

Harness the power of the placebo

Do you believe? If so, you just might feel better. The power of belief, expectation, and hope can play a dramatic role in your wellness. This is called the placebo effect, and it involves your mind's ability to alter physical symptoms, such as pain, anxiety, depression, and fatigue.

A placebo is a harmless pill, medicine, or procedure given to a patient in place of traditional medicine or therapy. The amazing thing is some people, unaware they are taking a placebo, actually start feeling better. Many doctors think these people get better because they expect to.

While placebos are most often linked to conditions that don't have exact causes — like irritable bowel syndrome — or illnesses where the symptoms are subjective — like headaches or dizziness — history has proven placebos can have real and beneficial effects in many situations.

- Asthma sufferers using a placebo inhaler in a 2011 study were able to breathe more easily.
- German researchers discovered people using a placebo cream on their skin not only reported feeling less pain when heat was applied to their arms, but actually had less pain signaling through the nerves in their spinal cords.
- Hotel workers who were told they were getting a good workout at their jobs lost weight and body fat and lowered

their blood pressure. Women who did the same work but didn't associate it with exercise showed no changes.

- Students participating in a sleep study were connected to a bogus machine that supposedly measured sleep quality. The next day, those who were told their deep sleep had been above average performed better on attention and memory tests than those told their sleep quality had been poor. This phenomenon is called placebo sleep.
- Antidepressants were the third top-selling drug of 2013, with one in particular reaping over $1 billion in sales in just three months. And yet, an analysis of more than 2,000 clinical trials of antidepressants showed that half the participants who improved took a placebo.
- Placebos have also successfully treated angina, high blood pressure, gastric reflux, psoriasis, and anxiety.

Even the color of a medication can have an effect. Research shows that people expect blue or green pills to have a calming effect and red, yellow, or orange pills to have a stimulating effect. In one study, people were told they were taking either a sedative or a stimulant, but they were actually given pink or blue placebos. Twice as many people taking the blue pills reported drowsiness as those who took the pink pills.

All these examples highlight how fundamentally your mind and body are connected. Just remember that while the placebo effect has great healing potential, not everyone responds in the same way. But if you truly believe or expect a therapy to help you, and you do all that is expected of you during the treatment, you're more likely to experience some real benefit.

CAUTION

Beware — negative thoughts can harm your health

Just as you can experience the placebo effect and feel better, the exact opposite is also possible. The nocebo effect is when you take a sham treatment and feel worse. It's the power of your mind at work again — your physical body all tied up with your thoughts, beliefs, and expectations. This phenomenon:

- most often occurs in people who also respond positively to placebos.
- is more common if you are depressed, anxious, or obsessed about your health.
- is more likely if someone trustworthy implies you could experience pain or some other negative reaction after taking a medication.

Common nocebo symptoms are headache, nausea, dizziness, confusion, and drowsiness. But they can be more specific. For instance, in one study, asthma sufferers experienced difficulty breathing after using an inhaler they were told contained an irritant. In fact, it contained a harmless saline solution. In cases like these, even though no real drug is used, the side effects are very real.

Live positively to live well

"Gratitude," say Yale University researchers, "is one of life's most vitalizing ingredients." You may think it's simply feeling a warm glow when someone holds the elevator or gives you a compliment. But in fact, many experts believe gratitude is the linchpin of positive psychology, a branch of science studying the strengths and virtues that allow people to live healthy, meaningful lives.

More than basic thankfulness, gratitude is showing appreciation for kindness, and, most importantly, returning that kindness. In this way, gratitude can have a dramatically positive effect on your life and the lives of others. It strengthens relationships, an important factor in the happiness equation. And when you express gratitude, you inspire others to continue acting generously. In other words, you foster a continuous cycle of good behavior and gratitude.

Combine it with other constructive forms of thinking — like optimism, satisfaction, and hope — and you've got one big package of well-being wrapped up with a feel-good bow.

Heal with positive emotions. According to research, people who react to life events positively are less depressed, happier, and more satisfied with their lives. But there are other, critical ways these emotions are good for you. Having a positive attitude can mean you:

- have a lower risk of heart disease and, if you already have heart disease, better odds of living longer.
- are more likely to exercise, and thus reap all the benefits that come with an active lifestyle.
- have a reduced risk of stroke.
- find it easier to follow a healthy eating regimen.
- are better equipped to survive a traumatic event.
- have lower levels of the stress hormone cortisol and deal better with everyday anxieties.
- have reduced blood pressure.
- generally feel more alert, enthusiastic, determined, attentive, and energetic.
- experience a boost to your immune function, so you may suffer from fewer chronic conditions and recover more quickly from illness.

- will stay physically independent longer.
- sleep better.

Decide to be optimistic. Keep in mind, positive traits like gratitude do not always come naturally or easily. These are more often learned behaviors — you must consciously choose to be grateful or happy. This will, at first, require discipline. But the longer you practice, the more it will become second nature.

Here are 10 easy ways you can develop a lifesaving, positive attitude.

- Keep a gratitude journal. In it list all the good things that have happened to you today, this week, or this month.
- Spend time outdoors communing with nature.
- Bring to mind a nostalgic event — a time or occasion you associate with happy personal feelings. For even more of a feel-good boost, think about an event you are looking forward to.
- Volunteer. Just four hours a week may help fend off high blood pressure and make you feel better emotionally, one study reports.
- Spend your money on experiences you can share rather than on material things. Enjoying times with others creates a bond that's just plain good for you, body and soul.
- Listen to happy music.
- Write a letter of gratitude to someone in your life — and send it. Or simply create a journal entry about that person.
- Try to respond positively when it seems others are acting badly or showing anger.
- Decide you're going to "try" to be cheerful. It helps if you couple this with an outward, physical expression — smile, even if you don't feel like it.

- Perform some small act of kindness every week. Change it up. Don't do the same thing for the same people week after week. A variety of these good deeds seems to work best.

Forgiveness — the key to well-being

It sounds so easy — just let go. Let go of hurt feelings and resentment. Let go of bitterness and hostility. Sounds easy, sure, but it may be the hardest thing you'll ever do. Still, try.

Forgive others and you'll replace anger with joy. Forgive yourself and you'll feel like a weight has lifted from your shoulders. Do it, and you will be a happier and healthier person.

Yes, to forgive and forget may be easier said than done, but here's why and how to let go.

Forgive others. Nelson Mandela said, "Resentment is like drinking poison and then hoping it will kill your enemies." How true that your bad feelings don't hurt the other person at all. They only hurt you.

The longer you are unforgiving, the longer your body experiences stress and its damaging effects. Whenever you think or talk about the hurt or injustice, your blood pressure rises. Even if you try to focus on something else, if the resentment is still inside you, your heart doesn't recover.

Forgiveness, on the other hand, makes people feel like they are in control. Research shows it can lower blood pressure and heart rate, reduce stress levels, ease pain, and lessen your chance of illness. In fact, a study out of the University of Wisconsin-Madison showed that heart patients who received forgiveness counseling and learned to work through their grudges had considerably fewer heart symptoms, like angina, than those who didn't get the counseling.

It will also improve your relationships with others. People who forgive are apt to have more friends and longer marriages, feel better about themselves, and be less likely to suffer from depression.

You may find it easier to forgive someone if you're clear in your mind that forgiveness does not mean:

- you must reconcile or establish a relationship with that person.
- you'll be able to forget the wrong that was done to you.
- there will ever be a valid excuse or defense for what was done.
- you will receive an apology, compensation, or any sense of justice.

Forgive yourself. When you think you have done something wrong, you may feel guilty and ashamed. You may not believe you are worthy of forgiveness or happiness. This translates into stress, depression, and anxiety. Many people even stop taking care of themselves as they used to. Because of this, the potential health hazards of self-blame and regret are serious.

A recent study out of Brandeis University found self-compassion, or the ability to forgive yourself, protects against inflammation from stress and inflammation-related disease, like heart disease, cancer, and Alzheimer's disease.

Some experts believe as long as you're holding on to negative emotions, you can't experience positive ones. So by forgiving others or yourself, you not only dump everything that's harmful about unforgiveness, but you allow healthy, constructive feelings in. Remember, forgiveness is not something you do for other people. It is something you do for yourself so you can heal and move on.

Let it go. The road to forgiveness is different for each person, but here are some steps you can take that may help you get there.

- Acknowledge what happened. Recall the event as objectively as possible.
- Try a little empathy. This will be hard, but see if you can tell the story from the other person's point of view. If you are honest, you may be surprised what you discover.
- Visualize a life without this hurt or anger.
- Continuously remind yourself that others have forgiven far greater hurts. Recall times when you have been forgiven.
- Mentally wish your "enemy" well, even if you can't truly mean it at first. Keep it up, and, over time, your feelings may change.
- Stop telling your story of injustice. The more you repeat it, the more you dwell on it. And research shows, becoming overly preoccupied with life's negative events means you may never defeat them.

Find healing grace in prayer

Religion and health care have been intertwined for thousands of years. Monks, priests, shamans, and medicine men were all once healers as well as spiritual leaders for their communities — in many cases until the late 1800s, when Western medicine and religion truly separated. Today, doctors never ask about your spirituality. This may be a mistake, since an astonishing amount of scientific evidence links religion and well-being. There are three elements that usually define religion.

- Beliefs are what connect you to God or a higher power. They can bring comfort and meaning during difficult circumstances.
- Practices or rituals offer a structure for your relationship with God. Attending church regularly means social support that is so important to good health. And praying not only gives you a sense of control, but a way to calm and focus yourself.

- Behaviors that are accepted by the community of your religion, like honesty, fidelity, and fairness, can give you a moral compass to live by, reduce stress, and encourage healthy habits.

Here are four ways these dimensions of spirituality can keep you healthy.

Boost mental health. Most of the research on spirituality has to do with mental health. And, overwhelmingly, the results show practicing some type of religion helps people cope with illness, stress, and hardship.

Based on more than 3,000 studies spanning close to 140 years, researchers found that religious people were optimistic, happy, and felt they had meaning and some sense of control in their lives, when compared to people who were not religious. That also meant they were less likely to suffer from depression, anxiety, and other mental health issues. Many experts think it is a belief in God or a higher power that helps you battle negative emotions and the isolating effects of mental difficulties.

Prayer, specifically, is a healthy habit. A study of more than 1,000 members of the Presbyterian Church of the United States found that those who prayed more also reported a greater sense of well-being, experiencing less depression and anxiety. Those who prayed at least two times every day — 42 percent of the group — had the best mental health.

Reduce daily stress. Stress not only takes a toll on your emotions but can make you more susceptible to illness and early death. Having a sense of purpose, believing in a God that cares about you, feeling you are part of a supportive community, and practicing prayer all help you cope with the pressures of daily living.

Protect your heart. In developed countries, heart disease is the most common cause of both death and disability. But you may be protecting your heart every time you practice your spiritual beliefs. In fact, religion seems to have a greater beneficial effect on heart disease than any other illness, say researchers who looked at more than 100 studies on spirituality and death.

In a survey of close to 4,000 people, those who attended religious services regularly and prayed or studied the Bible were 40 percent less likely to have high blood pressure than infrequent churchgoers or Bible readers. Spending a few moments quietly relaxing, controlling your breathing and emotions, and handing your problems to a higher power could all be part of prayer's healing ability.

The psychological benefits of religion — positive emotions of happiness, optimism, well-being, and hope — affect your immune, inflammatory, endocrine, and autonomic functions, which, in turn, influence heart health. In addition, if you're part of a religious community, it often encourages you to take better care of your physical body — even teaching you to treat your body as a "temple of the Holy Spirit."

Strengthen your immune system. Stress is your immune system's worst enemy. When you feel stressed, your brain tells your body to pump out massive amounts of hormones that direct all focus to your heart rate, blood pressure, breathing, and other survival functions. Processes like your immune system are pretty much shut down. That means for the time you're under stress, your cells can't effectively fight bacteria and viruses. Control stress and you allow your immune system to do its job.

You've already learned that prayer and other aspects of a spiritual life do this on an emotional level. But there is evidence that prayer, which scientists often refer to as spiritual meditation, impacts your immune system on a biological level.

Be aware that even experts who report on the benefits of spirituality warn that anything can be taken too far. Don't use your religious beliefs as an excuse to avoid seeing a doctor or getting help for your physical or mental problems.

CAUTION

Trans fats sabotage your mental health

Having trouble staying positive and happy? Is it increasingly difficult to let go of your anger and forgive? Perhaps that microwave popcorn or chocolate chip cookie is to blame. Or at least the trans fats in them are.

This unhealthy fat is produced during a process called hydrogenation, when hydrogen is added to vegetable oil to help it remain solid at room temperature. It's most commonly found in shortening, margarine, snack foods, store-bought baked goods, and fried foods in restaurants.

A recent study showed the more trans fats people ate, the more they suffered from impatience, irritability, and aggression.

Although the Food and Drug Administration has declared war on trans fat and is working to require food makers to gradually phase out its use, you can still find it in many products. And that's bad news for your mental and physical health.

For a happier you, avoid trans fats by eating whole, fresh foods instead of prepackaged ones.

9 reasons laughter is the best medicine

It may sound like a funny way to stay healthy, but laughter is no joke. Research shows that laughing can seriously improve your health. Find out how chuckling, giggling, cackling, and guffawing may help you live longer.

Improve blood flow. Loosen up with laughter, and your blood vessels will do the same. That's what researchers at the University of Maryland School of Medicine discovered.

In one study, when people watched scenes from a funny movie, their blood vessels expanded, improving blood flow. On the other hand, watching stressful scenes from a dramatic film caused blood vessels to constrict, impeding blood flow. The contrast between the conditions was stark, with a 30- to 50-percent difference in blood vessel diameter. Researchers noted that the improvement is similar to the beneficial effects of aerobic exercise or the use of statins.

A pair of studies at the University of Texas yielded similar results. In both studies, participants watched 30 minutes of either a comedy or a disturbing documentary. Those who watched the comedy had improved "arterial compliance," the amount of blood that flows through your arteries at a given time. That's important because decreased arterial compliance has been linked to high blood pressure and heart disease.

In the other study, the comedy watchers' blood vessels dilated by 21 percent, while the blood vessels of those who watched the documentary constricted by 18 percent. Constricted blood vessels can contribute to high blood pressure. Most encouraging, the positive effects of laughter lingered even 24 hours later.

Of course, you don't have to watch comedies to laugh. Japanese researchers found that "laughter yoga," which combines breathing exercises with laughter, helped lower blood pressure.

Elevate good cholesterol. High cholesterol is no laughing matter — but laughing may help your heart by boosting levels of HDL, or good cholesterol.

In a yearlong study of people with type 2 diabetes, high blood pressure, and high cholesterol, those who watched 30 minutes of funny movies or sitcoms each day in addition to their standard treatment reaped the benefits. After just two months, their HDL levels improved. After fourth months, they also lowered blood levels of certain inflammatory chemicals associated with heart disease.

Lower blood sugar. If you have diabetes, you need to take care of your heart — but don't forget about your blood sugar. Luckily, laughter comes in handy for that, too. A Japanese study found that laughing may help you sidestep unhealthy spikes in blood sugar that can follow meals. Laughter seems to work by sparking changes in genes that regulate blood glucose, thus improving glucose tolerance.

Ease pain. Sometimes you might laugh till it hurts. But a little silliness can also help soothe your pain. Laughing may work by contracting and relaxing certain muscles or just by providing a pleasant distraction. But a recent British study sheds more light on what makes laughter such good medicine.

Turns out that laughing triggers the release of endorphins, brain chemicals that act as natural painkillers. Researchers discovered that laughing actually boosts your tolerance for pain. It's the physical act of laughing itself that helps, so a hearty belly laugh or guffaw works better than a slight chuckle.

Boost your brainpower. "What is laughter?" could be the correct "Jeopardy" response to the clue "Best medicine for a better brain."

A recent Northwestern University study found that people performed better in a word association game after watching a stand-up comedy routine rather than news clips. MRI scans of those who watched the funny video showed increased activity in an area of the brain responsible for broadening attention. That's probably how they were suddenly able to find less obvious connections between words to solve the puzzles. Older studies have also suggested that humor improves memory.

Enhance your immune system. Laughter may be contagious, but it may also help you fight off sickness. A series of studies at Loma Linda University explored the effects of "mirthful laughter" on the immune system using blood samples. People who watched a humorous video for an hour boosted the activity of disease-fighting T cells and natural killer cells, which stave off tumors and viral infections.

Burn calories. Give your funny bone a workout, and you just might end up slightly slimmer. Like exercise, laughing burns calories — just not as many. Vanderbilt University researchers found that laughter boosted heart rate and energy expenditure by 10 to 20 percent. That's about the same rate as light clerical work, writing, or playing cards.

But a little laughter each day can add up. Researchers estimate that 15 minutes of genuine laughter each day can burn up to 40 calories. Over a year, that can mean a loss of more than 4 pounds.

Spark your appetite. Now here's the punch line — all that laughter can make you hungry. Loma Linda researchers found that laughter has the same appetite-stimulating effect as moderate physical exercise. Specifically, laughing changes the levels of hormones that regulate hunger. After watching a funny video, people had lower levels of leptin, which suppresses appetite, and higher levels of ghrelin, which stimulates hunger. This funny business can come in handy for older people who don't have much of an appetite and have difficulty exercising.

Squelch stress. When you're laughing, your worries disappear in a hurry. Laughter reduces levels of stress hormones like cortisol and epinephrine and helps you relax. That's important because stress can have a harmful effect on your health, contributing to high blood pressure, heart attack, stroke, memory loss, and other serious conditions.

Relax, recharge, renew

Stress — the secret cause of health problems

Your body works so well because it functions as a single organism. To paraphrase Matthew 6:3 — your left hand does, indeed, know what your right hand is doing. And that is all because of your autonomic nervous system (ANS), which connects your central nervous system to your internal organs. It is divided into the sympathetic nervous system, which mobilizes energy and resources during times of stress and arousal, and the parasympathetic nervous system, which conserves energy and resources during relaxed states.

This complicated, but elegant, network of nerves acts as a control system for most of the involuntary functions in your body — your heart rate and blood flow, digestion, breathing, and the production of hormones, saliva, mucus, perspiration, and urine. You don't have to think about these things. They just happen.

But sometimes they happen at the wrong time. Take stress, for example. It can come in handy in times of danger by preparing your body for action. An immediate threat, such as a charging lion, triggers the release of the stress hormone cortisol as well as the neurotransmitters dopamine, norepinephrine, and epinephrine — known collectively as catecholamines.

During this "fight or flight" response, your heart rate and blood pressure go up, your blood flow increases, your breathing speeds up, and your immune system gears up to deal with potential injuries. When the threat passes, everything returns to normal.

Or at least it should. The problem is that everyday pressures — including financial worries, relationship issues, health problems, job demands, and traffic jams — can trigger the same response, without much time to recover. This chronic stress takes its toll on both your physical and mental health.

Harms your heart. Experiencing stress can be as bad for your heart as smoking five cigarettes a day. You can blame much of the damage on the stress hormones that continuously flood your body when you're anxious. Your circulatory system stays on high alert for an extended period of time and, as you just learned, that means higher blood pressure and a faster heart rate. It also means your body produces more C-reactive protein, a marker of tissue inflammation that is linked to heart disease and other serious illnesses.

In addition, you behave differently when you're stressed, and many of these behaviors are just plain bad for your heart. For instance, when you're tense do you crave comfort food? Too many bowls of macaroni and cheese or chocolate chip ice cream will pack on the pounds, and that spells heart trouble by the spoonful.

Shrinks your brain. When you have trouble adapting to stress, it can lead to depression or anxiety. Scientists also say, over time, stress and depression damage brain cells. A 20-year University of Pittsburgh study found that chronic life stress led to a decrease in the volume of the hippocampus, a brain region essential for learning and memory.

Other studies have linked high levels of stress hormones to worse memory, focus, and problem-solving skills. That makes sense, because a barrage of stress hormones can shrink brain cells and disrupt connections between them.

Leads to belly fat. Emotional eating can be a heartbreaking cycle — you feel stressed, so you eat, then you gain weight and feel stressed, so you eat some more. On top of that, emotional eating rarely involves healthy food choices. You're drawn to calorie-dense foods, high in sugar and fat, that are designed to replenish your energy stores.

Unfortunately, modern stress doesn't involve running for your life from hungry predators. You are usually tense from work, relationships, or other emotional issues. So extra calories are just that — extra calories. Experts also say stress causes a shift in the balance of hormones in your body, triggering those calories to get stored as fat — particularly abdominal fat.

In one recent study, the eating habits of otherwise healthy women were evaluated during times of stress. The highly stressed group showed more emotional eating and greater belly fat than the low-stress group.

Disrupts your sleep. Difficulty sleeping is so closely related to stress that the National Institute of Mental Health lists it as one of the most basic signs you're suffering from this damaging condition. In fact, some experts say stress is the number one cause of insomnia. Surges of cortisol during times of stress create the opposite effect of everything your body needs to relax and sleep. Your heart beats faster, your mind races, and you feel extra alert.

Stress can be quite a menace. If yours becomes unmanageable, you may want to seek professional help. But first try the following amazingly easy, no-drug solutions.

Breathe in some peace of mind

Take a deep breath, count to 10, and feel your worries fall away. Well, that's how it's supposed to work. In reality, you may have to practice more control over your breathing, and do it for longer than a count of 10. But the basic idea holds — you can change the way you breathe to get control of your stress level. Doing that may well boost your immune system, which, in turn, may add years to your life.

Give your immunity a leg up. Your immune system gets revved up for a short time whenever you encounter a sudden stressful event. That reaction is your body getting ready to fight off infection — or maybe a grizzly bear.

But if the stress remains for a long period, you wear down your immunity and your ability to fight off that infection. Too much pressure on the system over time simply causes more wear and tear. The cells of your immune system, made to fight off foreign invaders like harmful bacteria and viruses, do not function as well after you suffer long-term stress. Seniors and people suffering from another illness are at even greater risk. That's why living with constant stress raises your chances of getting sick.

Change the way you breathe. You take about 14 to 16 breaths each minute while you are at rest. But when you are in a stressful situation, you tend to breathe faster as your lungs work to take in more oxygen as part of the fight or flight response.

Here's how deep breathing helps. When you breathe deeply, you work your diaphragm, the powerful sheet of muscle that separates your lungs from your stomach. Taking a deep breath lowers your diaphragm, pulling your lungs down with it and pressing against organs in your abdomen to make room for your lungs to expand as they fill with air. Then as you breathe out, your diaphragm presses up against your lungs, pushing out carbon dioxide. This kind of deep breathing engages what is called the "relaxation response." That is the opposite of the stress response.

Research shows that practicing deep-breathing exercises can lower your anxiety, stress, and depression while it increases your feelings of optimism. It's free and safe stress relief, and you can do it anywhere, at any time.

Get healthier and happier in 10 minutes

Here are 20 things you can do that will fill you with positive emotions, eliminate stress, and generally make you healthier. The best part — none takes more than 10 minutes.

1. Send a friendly email to a friend.
2. Read an inspirational quote and share it with someone.
3. Smile.
4. Say thank you to someone.
5. Give your mother, father, sister, or brother a call.
6. Ask a friend to join you for a healthy dinner.
7. Hug someone you love.
8. Don't nag.
9. Laugh out loud.
10. Go to bed one hour earlier than usual.
11. Put your favorite music on and sing.
12. Declutter one spot in your home or office.
13. Say no to one thing that compromises your personal goals.
14. Turn off the news.
15. Sit outside.
16. Play with a pet.
17. Light a scented candle.
18. Say a prayer for someone.
19. Write down one positive thing about your day.
20. Let go of one grudge.

Follow the path to stress relief. Find time to do these deep-breathing exercises several times each day, even if you don't feel especially stressed. First, inhale through your nose slowly and deeply, counting to 10. Be sure your stomach and abdomen expand, but your chest does not. Then, exhale through your nose slowly, also while you count to 10. Concentrate on counting and breathing through each cycle to quiet your mind. Repeat the cycle five to 10 times.

Get your muscles in on the action. You can add progressive muscle relaxation, especially if your goals include cutting stress, relaxing, and getting some very important sleep. Small studies have shown it may even help lower blood pressure. Here's how.

- Lie down and get comfortable. Don't cross your arms or legs.
- Be sure you continue breathing slowly.
- Tense one muscle group tightly while you count to 10. Then release that muscle group and move on to the next one.
- Begin with muscles at the top of your head, then move downward through muscle groups like your upper arms, lower arms, hands, thighs, calves, feet, and so on.
- Concentrate on how relaxed and heavy your muscles feel when they're released.

5 top stress-busting strategies

Everyone reacts to stress differently, so you need to choose the best relaxation technique for you. It must feel right and match your fitness level and lifestyle. Plus, you may need more than one strategy to keep you motivated and give you the best results.

Here are some simple ways to control stress. Try them and you just might live longer and happier.

Tune in to a tune. There's an Irish blessing that says, "May your heart be as light as a song." Well, the Irish may be on to something. Modern science is finding that a song may, indeed, lighten your heart.

Have you noticed that hearing a favorite song on the radio just seems to make you feel good? It actually is making you feel good. Listening to music can reduce stress, relieve depression and anxiety, lower blood pressure, decrease heart rate, manage pain, and generally improve your quality of life.

While you should listen to a style of music you like, researchers found cancer patients responded to different genres in different ways. Cheerful music, naturally, helped them feel happier and more optimistic. Heavy-metal music allowed some to release their anger and frustrations, while songs involving sounds of nature gave the patients a sense of strength and life. If you're Christian, listening to religious music — particularly gospel — may be the key to easing your tension.

While singing or bopping to the radio is an easy and affordable solution to stress, try any of the creative arts — such as creative writing, dance, drawing, or even playing a musical instrument — to reduce your anxiety and depression.

Get moving. Work out a little and work off that stress. Researchers are finding out that people who regularly exercise tend to feel good about themselves and often translate that into confidence and a sense of balance in their lives. That means the individual stresses of home and work don't bother them as much.

In one recent study out of the University of Maryland, people who took part in 30 minutes of moderate exercise were able to keep their cool under pressure afterward better than people who didn't exercise.

Not an exercise junkie? Then here's even better news for you. One of the best ways to wind down and let go of worries is to take a walk. There's a rhythm to it that's soothing, especially if you refuse to let your mind dwell on problems as you amble along. After all, the whole point is to let go of stress.

Try focusing, instead, on your breath, your feet hitting the ground, or simply the way your body feels and moves. Practice this focused walking for 10 minutes every day, and research shows you can reduce your stress and improve your quality of life. Among other things, walking like this gives you a chance to breathe deeply, which will clear your mind, slow your heart rate, lower your blood pressure, give you energy, and improve your mood.

If you walk outside, you'll reap even more benefits. Scientists have found walking in a forest or park boosts your immune function by increasing your body's natural killer cells. It also lowers levels of the stress hormone cortisol at the same time. Expand your focus to include the nature around you, and you may feel a sense of gratitude and well-being that melts away tension.

Find a distraction. Do you obsess over a problem? Is it hard to let go of a mistake? If you find your mind constantly circles the same territory, you're probably churning out high levels of stress hormones. A great way to let go of this stress is to distract yourself. Shift those mental gears and your cortisol levels will drop. Consider reading a book, doing a puzzle, or perhaps playing a game. Scientists even tested a smartphone app to help focus attention on positive cues. Find a distraction you enjoy that will truly occupy your mind.

Bond with someone. If there's one thing in particular that has cranked up your anxiety, try talking about it with someone who has similar feelings. Sarah Townsend, assistant professor of management and organization at the USC Marshall School of Business, calls this "emotional similarity." In a 2013 study, she found that people nervous about speaking in public had lower stress levels if they shared their feelings with a partner having the same fears.

And while you may not have to agree on everything, if you're in a loving, supportive relationship with someone, you're likely to have lower levels of stress and anxiety in your day-to-day life.

Take a supplement. Multivitamins have come under fire lately with many experts questioning their usefulness. And, yes, the jury may still be out on whether or not they can prevent chronic disease. But evidence shows a good vitamin and mineral supplement can give you the mental energy you need to manage stress, fight fatigue, and boost your mood.

In addition, you may want to include a fish oil supplement as part of your daily regimen. Researchers out of Michigan found that people taking this omega-3 fatty acid did not have as strong a fight-or-flight response to stress as people taking olive oil.

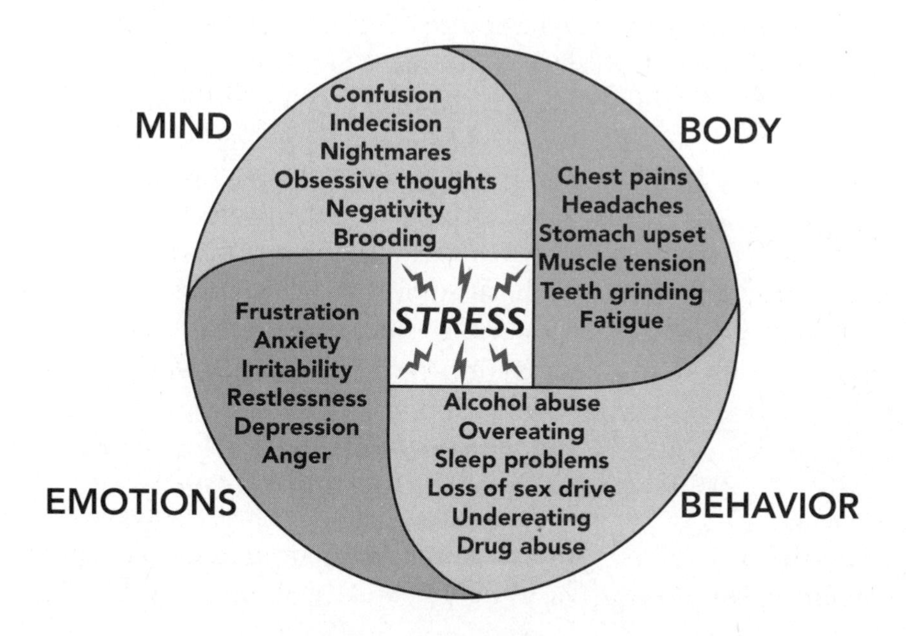

Negative effects of stress

Sleep right to save your life

Sidestep sleeping pill dangers

Getting the rest and relaxation you need is not a luxury — it's a necessity for long-term health. Cut back on sleep by even an hour or two and you've put your body under stress. This can trigger the release of too much adrenaline, cortisol, and other stress hormones.

In addition, depression and fatigue are part of a dangerous cycle. According to the National Sleep Foundation, people with insomnia have 10 times the risk of developing depression compared with those who sleep well. And when you're depressed, you're four times more likely to develop fatigue. Dr. Tim Hayden, a family doctor in Tennessee, even says, "The number one cause of fatigue in my practice is depression." That's why so many people are desperate for a good night's sleep.

But sleeping pills are not the answer to these troublesome nights. You might think the dangerous side effects — short-term memory loss, headaches, daytime fatigue, nausea, and dizziness — as well as the risk of dementia and even death, would be discouragement enough. Still, almost 9 million Americans use sleep aids regularly — seniors, more than any other age group.

And that's cause for concern because these drugs are more dangerous in the elderly. The older you are, the more likely it is you'll experience side effects and reactions with sleeping pills. Plus, your body takes longer to purge the drug from your system so the effects can last for a long time.

If you must take a sleep aid, follow these steps to protect yourself:

- Take the lowest dose possible or halve the dose.
- Take them for the shortest amount of time possible.
- Don't drink alcohol while taking sleep aids.
- Don't drive, even the morning after.
- Talk to your doctor about alternatives.

Take these smart steps to sounder sleep

Frustrated over yet another night of tossing and turning? Break the cycle with these natural ways to get to sleep — and stay asleep all night long.

Establish a regular bedtime routine. Go to bed at roughly the same time every night, and wake up at the same time every morning. You may be tempted to sleep in on the weekends, but resist that temptation and stick to a schedule. Also plan some time for a relaxing activity before bedtime, like reading or listening to music, to help you wind down. But avoid pursuits like watching television or working on the computer just before bed. The lights from their bright screens can leave you too pumped up to get to sleep.

Avoid naps. You may think a midafternoon siesta will help you make it to bedtime, but a nap may do more harm than good. Sleeping during the day — especially in the late afternoon — can disrupt your body's natural sleep cycle and make it harder to fall asleep at night.

Don't exercise too close to bedtime. Physical activity during the day is a great way to get your body ready for sleep at night. One study found that exercise works as well for inducing sleep as taking a benzodiazepine prescription sleeping pill. Practicing yoga is especially good, because it involves meditation, deep breathing, and movements focusing on stretching and balance.

But don't exercise several hours before bed. Doing this can rev up your body and your mind, making it hard to relax in preparation for sleep.

Enjoy a hot bath. Take it about one or two hours before bed. Besides being relaxing, a bath will alter your body's core temperature, making it easier to fall asleep and sleep continuously through the night. Your body temperature tends to drop after you get out of a hot bath, mimicking what happens as your body gets ready for sleep.

Keep your bedroom cool. Experts say the ideal temperature for sleep is 60 to 72 degrees Fahrenheit. Lowering your body's temperature can bring on sleep, so it makes sense to aim for a feeling of coolness in the bedroom.

If menopause is making you wake up overheated in the middle of the night, pay attention to your bed coverings. Avoid that big quilt and use just a sheet instead. Also consider clothing made to keep you cool, like pajamas made from bamboo, which has great wicking ability. You may also want to turn on a fan in the room to boost air circulation, or even set the fan to blow across a pan of ice cubes to keep you cool.

Adjust your sleep position. How you curl up with your pillow at night can mean the difference between a peaceful evening and one that leaves you restless and with aching joints.

- Sleeping on your back can be a good choice if you suffer from back pain. Just place a pillow under your knees to keep pressure off your spine and to eliminate any arch in your back.
- Side sleepers need a firm pillow to avoid neck strain. Also, bend your knees, and place a pillow between them to protect your back and keep the natural curve in your spine.
- Don't sleep on your stomach if you have knee or neck pain, or suffer from plantar fasciitis. This position places pressure on your kneecaps, forces your neck into a stressed position, and causes your feet to point, which can cramp the muscles.

Don't watch the clock. Obsessing over the time just makes it harder to sleep. Having a bad attitude about your sleeplessness makes it worse. If you find yourself awake in the middle of the night, try to avoid these repeated negative thoughts — "I'm not getting enough sleep so I'll feel terrible tomorrow," "I hate it when I can't sleep," and "I'm angry about my insomnia."

Instead, change the way you think about your wakefulness, and trade those negative thoughts for positive ones — "I've had sleepless nights before, and I made it through just fine," "I'm probably getting some rest just lying here quietly," or "It's nice and quiet this time of the night." These positive thoughts will help you relax more than counting the hours until your alarm will sound.

Target sleep problems with better nutrition

Don't sacrifice your health when you're desperate for sleep. Try a few simple changes to your diet instead. There are specific foods proven to target sleep problems and boost your mood. After all, wouldn't you rather eat than pop pills? Put the right foods on your plate, and spend more quality time with your head on the pillow.

Choose cherries. Loaded with melatonin — a natural hormone that helps "shut off" your wakeful brain, improves the quality of sleep, and shortens the time needed to fall asleep — cherries could be the perfect bedtime snack.

While a handful of cherries a day should provide all the melatonin you need, you can also buy melatonin supplements. Researchers at the Massachusetts Institute of Technology (MIT) found a standard dose of about 3 milligrams (mg) overloads the melatonin receptors in your brain to the point they stop working. One-tenth of that amount — or just 0.3 mg — is enough to help you fall asleep and maintain better quality sleep.

Make room for magnesium. High levels of this mineral may help you fall asleep faster and sleep more soundly. Good sources include nuts, legumes, whole grains, dark leafy greens, and seafood.

Count on carbohydrates. An Australian study found that starchy carbohydrates eaten four hours before bedtime help people fall asleep faster. That's because they may boost levels of tryptophan and serotonin, two brain chemicals involved in sleep. Although the study used jasmine rice, you can try other types of carbohydrates that rank high on the glycemic index, which measures how quickly foods raise your blood sugar. Good options include mashed potatoes, bagels, saltine or Graham crackers, French bread, pretzels, and rice cakes.

Trim the fat. Several studies show that fatty foods give you a fat chance for a good night's sleep.

- Chinese men and women who slept less than seven hours a night ate more fat than those who slept seven to nine hours a night.
- An Israeli study of mice found that a high-fat diet affects the body clock, disrupting the sleep cycle.

- According to Brazilian researchers, total fat intake and fat intake at dinner negatively affect sleep patterns.

Lay off evening snacks. High-calorie, late-night snacks can mean you'll have a fitful night. In fact, simply eating too many calories during the day may lead to disrupted sleep.

Eliminate energy drinks. These products contain lots of caffeine — up to 141 mg per serving, more than an 8-ounce cup of coffee — and can lead to elevated blood pressure and heart rate. They're also loaded with sugar, sodium, and calories — often 200 or more per serving. Too much caffeine can cause increased heart rate, restlessness, anxiety, and nausea, as well as sleep deprivation. Worse, you may not know how much caffeine you're getting because the label doesn't always show this information.

Prevent a drowsy driving accident

Getting behind the wheel when you haven't had a good night's sleep is dangerous for you and everyone else on the road, yet more than half of all drivers have done it. No one plans to nod off while driving, but it's more likely to happen if you slept less than six hours the night before, or if you snore.

The National Sleep Foundation says the following are signs you, or the driver in your car, need to stop and take a rest.

- blurry vision, frequent blinking, or drooping eyelids
- trouble keeping your head up
- yawning
- feeling as if you're driving in a trance
- missing exits or traffic signs

- drifting from your lane, tailgating, or hitting a shoulder rumble strip
- restlessness or irritability

So now that you know the warning signs of fatigue — you must heed them. Here's what to do to make sure you don't fall asleep at the wheel.

Bring a friend. You're more likely to experience a drowsy driving crash if you're traveling alone. Have someone else in the car with you to help you stay awake and to watch for signs of fatigue.

Stop driving. Pull off as soon as possible to a rest area, restaurant, or hotel.

Take a nap. You only need to sleep for 15 to 20 minutes. More than that and you'll be too groggy to drive right away.

Consume some caffeine. It takes about 30 minutes for caffeine to enter your bloodstream, so plan ahead. Remember, you can get an eye-popping dose from soft drinks, tea, energy drinks, and even tablets or chewing gum. One cup of coffee can have as much as 200 milligrams of caffeine.

Switch drivers. Let a passenger take over the driving.

In addition, be careful about taking allergy and pain medications, tranquilizers, alcohol, and sleep aids. They can stay in your system far longer than you might think and can make you drowsy even the next day.

Wake up to the signs of sleep apnea

Eight out of 10 people with sleep apnea don't even know they have it. That's downright dangerous, considering you actually stop breathing when you have an apnea attack. Your windpipe gets blocked and you wake up gasping for air — sometimes hundreds of times a night. This start-stop breathing puts you at greater risk for stroke and heart disease.

It might not be easy to tell if you suffer from sleep apnea, but it's more likely if you're a heavy snorer. Experts have pieced together several clues to help you figure out if you have a problem.

Look for telltale sounds. One of the best ways to uncover sleep apnea is to listen for its distinctive noises. At first, an attack sounds just like the typical rattling snore. But without warning, you start to gag and choke, as you struggle to breathe. After several moments, you catch your breath and return to snoring like nothing happened. Ask your loved ones if they've heard this pattern during the night. Or, if you sleep alone, tape yourself for a few nights, and see if you hear it.

Be mindful of morning headaches. In a recent study from Dartmouth University, two-thirds of people who frequently had morning headaches also had sleep apnea. And eight out of 10 headache sufferers who also snored turned up with the sleep disorder. Sleep apnea seems to cause these headaches by cutting off oxygen to your brain, so it's important to treat the problem and get your breathing back to normal.

Keep an eye on cluster headaches. If your headaches come at night, that might be another clue, particularly if they're cluster headaches. These excruciating headaches that pierce one side of your head could be another symptom of sleep apnea's oxygen cutoff. Cluster attacks usually wake you up in the middle of the night, but they can strike in the morning, too.

Count your trips to the toilet. Stumbling to the bathroom late at night is not always a side effect of getting older. It could mean you have sleep apnea. A small study at the University of Alabama at Birmingham found a strong association between sleep apnea and nocturia, the urge to urinate at night.

Make sure it's not menopause. Twice as many postmenopausal women have sleep apnea as do premenopausal women. If you are postmenopausal and spot one of the other sleep apnea signals, you have a doubly good reason to talk with your doctor. She could recommend treatments geared just for you, like hormone replacement therapy (HRT).

If you suspect you have sleep apnea for any of these reasons, start your recovery by trying one of these simple lifestyle changes.

- Lose weight.
- Avoid alcohol and other sedatives before bedtime.
- Quit smoking.
- Sleep on your side instead of your back.

At the same time, talk with your doctor about the best way to proceed. Since sleep apnea is a potentially dangerous condition, you may need to be tested in a sleep center for an accurate diagnosis.

3 treatment options for sleep apnea sufferers

The gold standard for treating sleep apnea — the Continuous Positive Airway Pressure (CPAP) machine — can be difficult to use. As a result, many people don't stick with them. Fortunately, they aren't the only solution. Three exciting new developments may ease breathing and quiet snoring with less hassle.

Give your mouth a workout. Sixteen people with moderate sleep apnea gave their mouths a workout using tongue, soft palate, and throat exercises for 30 minutes every day. After three months, they were breathing easier, sleeping better, snoring less often and more quietly, and feeling more awake during the day, compared to sufferers who didn't do the exercises.

In obstructive sleep apnea, your upper airway collapses while you sleep, cutting off your breathing and waking you up. The researchers behind this study spent eight years developing exercises specifically to help stop this collapse. You may be able to learn them, too, by finding a speech therapist familiar with them. Ask your sleep doctor to recommend one.

Explore dental options. Oral appliances can now be used as the first line of treatment for mild to moderate sleep apnea, according to the American Academy of Sleep Medicine. But a new study suggests one mouthpiece may work for people with severe apnea, too.

Texas researchers tried the Thornton Adjustable Positioner (TAP) device in people who couldn't handle the traditional CPAP. "What we found was that many of our patients with moderate to severe sleep apnea were not adhering to standard treatment with a CPAP machine," says Paul McLornan, assistant professor in the Department of Prosthodontics at the University of Texas Dental School. Fewer than half were actually using their CPAPs, so researchers looked for another way to treat this condition.

The TAP is much smaller and fits right into your mouth. It pulls your lower jaw forward, keeping your airway open while you sleep. People in the study wore it every night, and, according to McLornan, it really worked. "We saw patients who began the study with severe sleep apnea end the study with very mild or no sleep apnea. They reported sleeping better and feeling more rested in the morning and altogether healthier." In fact, studies show people have better long-term success with oral appliances than with the standard surgery for sleep apnea, called UPPP.

The TAP isn't your only option. Other mouthpieces, such as the Dynamax, may treat mild to moderate apnea. Whichever one you choose, you'll need a dentist or orthodontist to make and fit you with it. Keep in mind, though, that oral appliances usually work best if you sleep on your back or stomach, not on your side.

Ask about implants. Pillar palatal implants mainly treat snoring, but they can also help mild to moderate sleep apnea. They're done in your doctor's office using local anesthesia. He will insert three short pieces of polyester string into the soft palate of your mouth to keep it from moving at night. Research shows it works as well as UPPP but with much less pain and a faster recovery.

The most important thing is to find something that works for you, whether it's a CPAP, dental appliance, or implant. Left untreated, obstructive sleep apnea contributes to heart attacks, coronary artery disease, high blood pressure, gastroesophageal reflux disease (GERD), and congestive heart failure. Plus, it shaves about 20 years off your life.

TAP Device for Mild Sleep Apnea

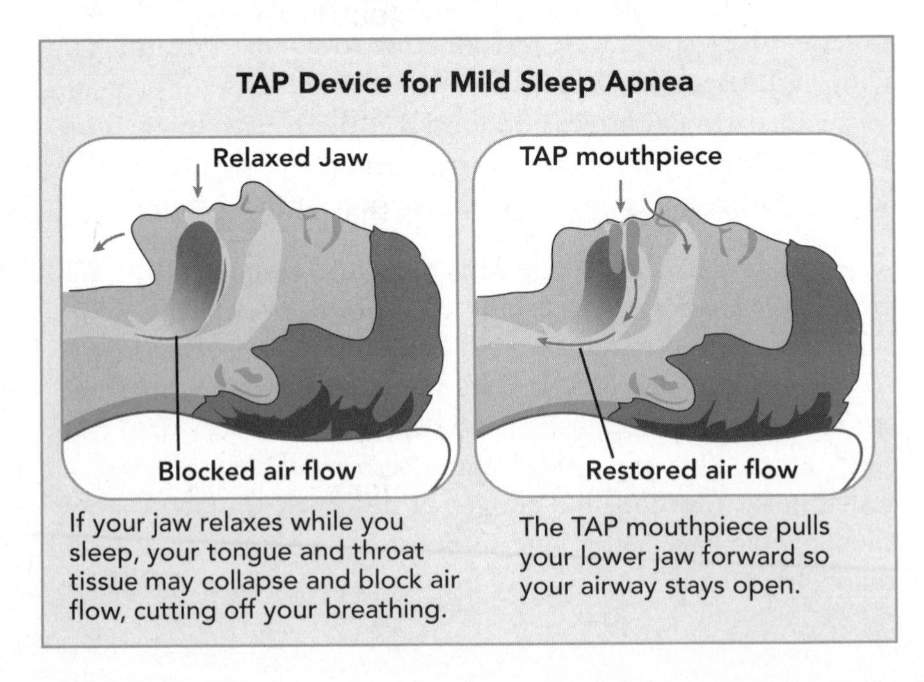

If your jaw relaxes while you sleep, your tongue and throat tissue may collapse and block air flow, cutting off your breathing.

The TAP mouthpiece pulls your lower jaw forward so your airway stays open.

Step 2: Eat to heal

You are what you eat

Food. Just the word summons an image, perhaps a memory, even an emotion. And rest assured, it means something different to every person.

Thank goodness for that. It's our diversity that means we have choices in our menus and supermarkets. Besides, who would want to eat the exact same thing every meal, every day?

But while food can range from hot dogs to Beef Wellington, take-out to five-star, that very diversity means you have the opportunity to make some exceptionally bad choices. Add to the mix your own complex tangle of history, culture, personality, and life experiences, and you have one big stew of a dietary dilemma.

So what should food mean to you? Let's start with the fundamentals. We all eat to live. And that's the point, really. Despite the seasonings and sauces, the garnish and ganache, it all comes down to sustenance. Without food you die.

But when you live to eat, you can die, too. Food without a healthy dose of nutritional sense can be fatal. For example, 36 percent of Americans over age 20 are obese. Twenty million women and 10 million men suffer from a dangerous eating disorder at some time in their life. And nearly every person in America gets more salt than they should, contributing to up to 40 percent of all cases of high blood pressure. If only they knew how easy it is to make smarter food choices.

Think of it this way. You would never pour any random liquid into your car's gas tank. So why would you fill your body with a haphazard assortment of fuel? Take some time to learn about the basic components of food — protein, carbohydrates, fiber, fats, vitamins, minerals, and phytochemicals. Learn to read food labels for sodium content and hidden calories in order to sidestep life-threatening disease. Start to understand nutritional building blocks, and you can assemble a menu that will satisfy not only your body but your soul as well.

Food should mean health, strength, and vitality. It should also mean enjoyment and comfort. So while your family, friends, beliefs, and culture all play a role in the foods you choose, let good information further guide you to a longer, healthier, more productive life.

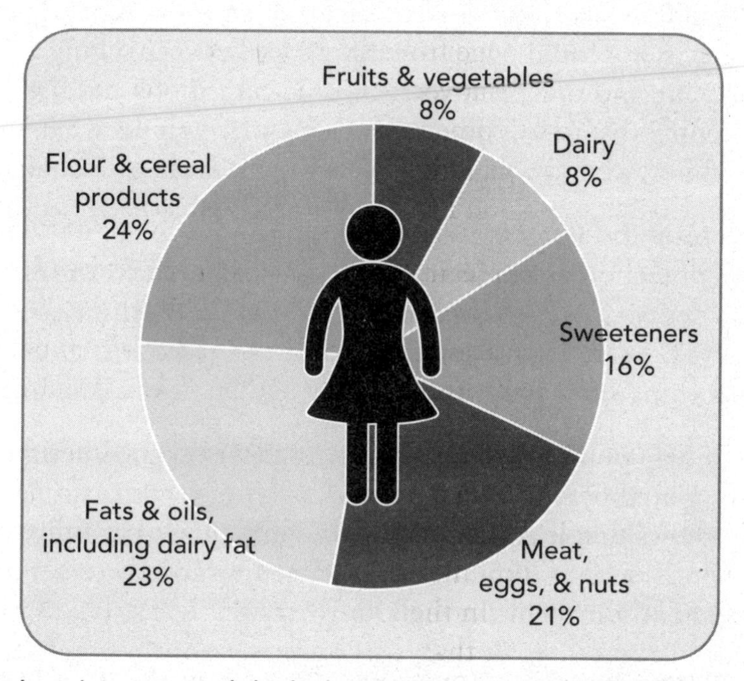

Americans eat and drink about 2,569 calories a day. As you can see, most of these come from unhealthy sources.

Food smarts: heroes to zeroes

Your food choices: 6 ways to turn bad into good

Every day you're faced with food choices. And since you eat well over 1,000 meals a year — that's a lot of choices. What drives your decisions could mean the difference between a long, healthy life and one filled with chronic conditions and life-threatening diseases. Learn more about why you eat what you eat and how you can make simple — but effective — changes.

Taste tops the list. Not surprisingly, taste is the number one reason you choose the foods you eat. After all, who can resist sugary sweets, salty snacks, and high-fat fare? Try this easy fix the next time you crave something salty — reach for 10 baked tortilla chips and a half cup of salsa, a low-fat, low-cal alternative.

And to help your young grandchildren develop good eating habits, give them healthy treats instead of sugary snacks. One study shows that if children are frequently offered healthy foods — even those they don't like — they're more likely to get used to them and eat them throughout their life.

Price must be nice. Some people think they can't afford to eat healthy. A recent survey by the International Food Information Council found that cost is the second most-important factor people look at in deciding what to eat. But consider this — an adult can satisfy fruit and vegetable recommendations from the *Dietary Guidelines for Americans* for an average cost of $2 to $2.50 daily. That's less than a bag of potato chips.

Convenience is key. A drive-thru or ready-to-eat meal beats cooking over a hot stove any day, especially if you're juggling work, children, and activities. But those foods aren't always the most nutritious. Satisfy your craving for convenience by freezing leftovers for a later meal or ordering a healthy take-out dish of sautéed chicken and vegetables.

Habits are hard to break. If you feast on bacon or pork sausage for breakfast every morning or can't pass up dessert after dinner every night, you've developed a food habit — and regrettably, not a good one. Studies show that new habits can take 10 weeks or longer to form. Start small, like eating turkey bacon for breakfast or a piece of fruit for dessert. Give yourself the freedom to splurge every now and then.

Regional fare rules. In the South, it's biscuits and gravy. Up North, it's buffalo wings. No matter where you grew up or where you live now, regional cuisine is hard to pass up. Keep the high fat and fried foods to a minimum. And try to make healthy substitutions, like fresh peaches instead of peach cobbler.

Comfort foods dominate plates. For some, it's a big bowl of ice cream. For others, a plate full of fried chicken. No matter how sad or stressed out you feel, emotional eating can lead to overeating and obesity. Learn to manage your emotions by taking a walk, talking to a friend, or doing something productive. Quench your craving for comfort foods occasionally, not daily.

A host of other reasons, from medical conditions to social engagements, can drive your food decisions. Whatever the reason, make it your goal to blend nutrient-rich meals into your daily diet, and you'll be on your way to a healthier life.

Pack your day with calories that pay off

You may think of calories as an enemy because the more you eat, the more pounds you pack on. But if you're smart about the foods you pick, you'll benefit from those calories by giving your body the healthy nutrients it needs.

Simply put, a calorie is a unit of energy — the energy released from fats, proteins, and carbohydrates. These units of energy are so tiny that it takes 1,000 of them to make up one kilocalorie, which is the technical name for the calories you eat. For instance, a medium-sized apple contains 95 kilocalories, but to keep things simple, it's labeled as 95 calories. That number represents how much energy your body gets from eating it. Carbohydrates and proteins contain four calories per gram while fat contains nine calories per gram.

So how many calories do you need each day? That depends on a number of things, including age, gender, and activity level. You'll need a different amount if you're trying to lose weight compared to maintaining it. And the number of calories you need to maintain your weight changes as you get older. The chart below from the USDA Center for Nutrition Policy and Promotion can help you determine your optimum daily calories.

	Male			Female		
Age	Sedentary	Moderately active	Active	Sedentary	Moderately active	Active
41-45	2,200	2,600	2,800	1,800	2,000	2,200
46-50	2,200	2,400	2,800	1,800	2,000	2,200
51-55	2,200	2,400	2,800	1,600	1,800	2,200
56-60	2,200	2,400	2,600	1,600	1,800	2,200
61-65	2,000	2,400	2,600	1,600	1,800	2,000
66-70	2,000	2,200	2,600	1,600	1,800	2,000
71-75	2,000	2,200	2,600	1,600	1,800	2,000
76+	2,000	2,200	2,400	1,600	1,800	2,000

Along with the number of calories in a food, you need to pay attention to the type of nutrients it has, which you can find by reading nutrition labels. Nutrition experts call foods rich in nutrients relative to the number of calories "nutrient dense." Foods with lots of calories but little nutrition are called "calorie dense." Why is this important to know? After all, if you eat the same number of calories daily to maintain your weight, does it matter where those calories come from? It does if you want to live a long, healthy life. Nutritionists recommend a diet packed with nutrient-dense meals and snacks to stay healthy.

Compare the two breakfast meals below. Each contains about 550 calories. The first meal includes two boiled eggs, two slices of Canadian bacon, one cantaloupe wedge, one cup of oatmeal, and an 8-ounce glass of orange juice. Meal number two is a homemade biscuit with a 2-ounce sausage patty.

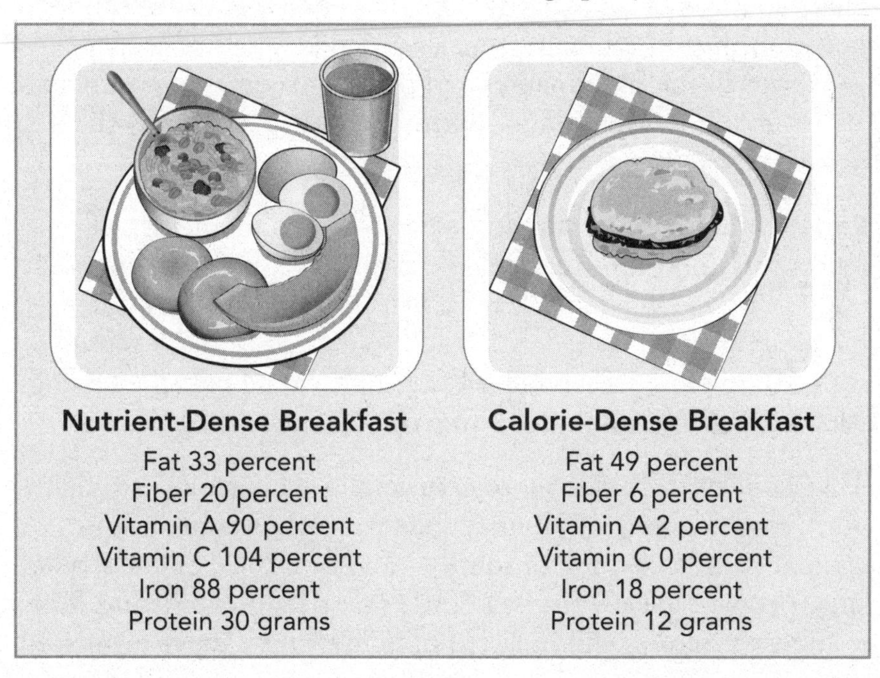

Even though each breakfast contains a similar number of calories, you can see how much they differ nutritionally. The sausage biscuit is loaded with fat but few nutrients. The egg breakfast is brimming with fiber, vitamins and minerals. Plus, nutrient-dense foods typically contain a lot of water and fiber, making them bulkier and more filling. All these benefits make the nutrient-dense egg breakfast a healthier, more satisfying choice.

New food label cuts the confusion

You no longer have to be a nutrition expert to read the hidden messages on a food label. Thanks to the Food and Drug Administration (FDA), the newly revised Nutrition Facts label on all foods will be easier to read and understand. Plus, shoppers can rest assured that the updated information is based on the latest dietary research.

A food label is like an atlas — it contains information that can guide you from an unhealthy lifestyle to one filled with sound nutrition. Just like a map, you can use food labels to prepare your trips to the supermarket and plan your meals to ensure you arrive at your destination — optimal health. Here's how the new label will help.

Ends confusion over serving size. New requirements will reflect the amount of food people actually eat today as opposed to 20 years ago when labels were first introduced. For instance, manufacturers typically labeled a 20-ounce soda as 2.5 servings with 110 calories per serving. Most people would miss the servings per container and think the entire soda contained 110 calories.

That's one of the hidden messages you'll no longer have to figure out. From now on, a 20-ounce soda will list its entire calorie content — 275 calories for some — and be labeled as one serving, since people typically drink a bottle that size in one sitting. The number of calories will be listed in bold using a larger print size.

Makes nutrition data easier to read. The percentage of daily values will shift to the left of the label to help shoppers calculate nutrient information more easily. The label will continue to include the daily value percentages for iron and calcium. It will add nutritional data for vitamin D and potassium because many Americans don't get enough of these critical nutrients.

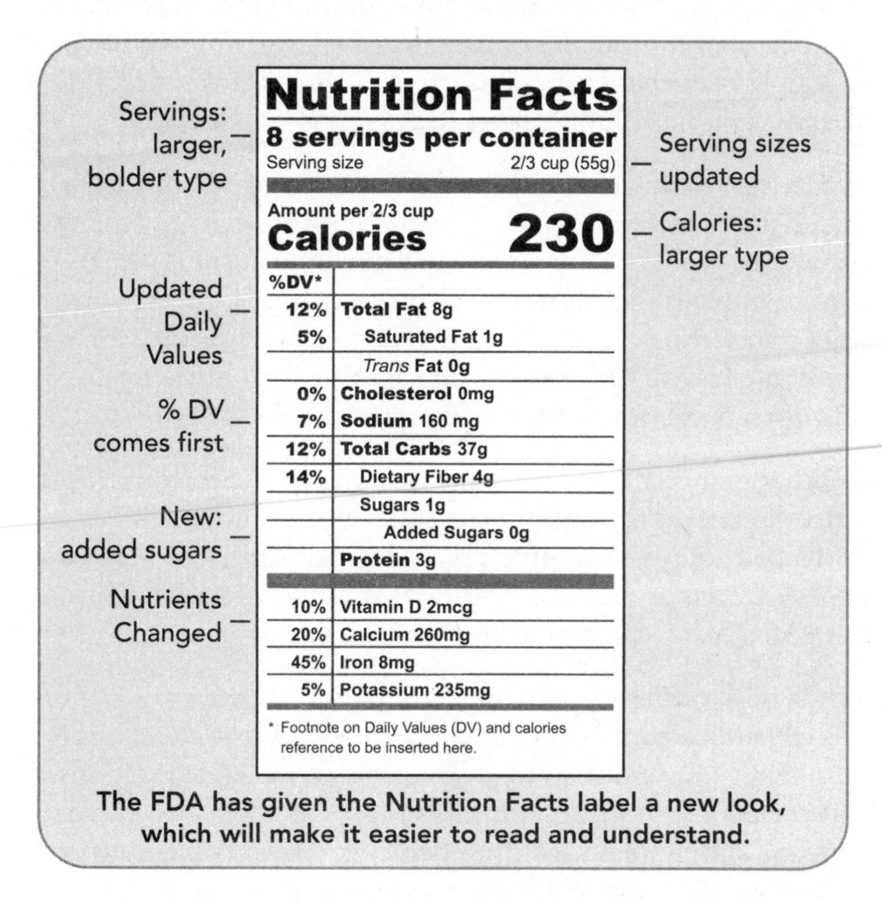

The FDA has given the Nutrition Facts label a new look, which will make it easier to read and understand.

Highlights added sugar. You won't be fooled by long, complicated sugar names any longer. In the past, manufacturers listed the scientific names of added sugars, and you had no way of knowing how much the product contained. The new food labels will list the total amount of added sugars in grams. While added sugar and naturally occurring sugar are similar chemically, foods loaded with added sugar deliver little to no nutrients. So if your favorite cereal has 10 grams of added sugar, you'll know it's not the healthiest choice.

Should science tinker with your food?

You've seen the phrase "Non GMO" on food products and wonder what it means. Or maybe you've heard your favorite vegetable is a genetically modified organism and wonder if it's a science experiment gone awry. Rest assured — it's not.

When a scientist tinkers with the DNA of a plant, animal, or insect, and inserts it into a food crop to improve it in some way, the altered plant is a genetically modified organism (GMO). One example is the vitamin-enriched tomato. Scientists created it by transferring a beta-carotene gene from carrots into the cells of tomato leaves. The tomato, already ripe with nutrients, is now even more nourishing.

Another example is the Hawaiian papaya. In the early 1990s, a virus threatened to wipe out the tropical fruit, but scientists developed a virus-resistant crop. Today, 80 percent of Hawaii's papaya crop is genetically modified. Without this GMO plant, the Aloha State's papaya plantations would not have survived.

While both of these examples seem harmless, critics say GMOs can jeopardize your health. They believe scientists could create a crop that's resistant to antibiotics or triggers allergic reactions. But the Food and Drug Administration says there's no cause for concern, stating that GMOs undergo extensive evaluations and must meet the same requirements as normally bred plants.

As the debate continues, you can avoid or limit GMOs if you're uneasy about their long-term effects.

- Look for packages with the Non GMO Project Verified seal or the USDA certified organic label.
- Choose whole foods over processed since 70 percent of processed foods contain at least one GMO ingredient.
- If you buy processed foods, avoid items with corn or soy additives, which are more likely to be genetically modified.

Vitamins and minerals: how much is enough?

Learning how much of each nutrient you need daily can seem like rocket science. And in many ways, it is a science. But it's an easy one to digest with the help of Dietary Reference Intakes or DRIs.

Established by a group of researchers in the United States and Canada, DRIs include Recommended Dietary Allowances (RDAs) and Adequate Intakes (AIs) for almost every nutrient imaginable.

RDA levels are based on scientific research. They tell you how much of a nutrient most healthy people of a particular age group and gender should get each day. AIs are set when scientists have too little data to establish an RDA value.

As you learn more about DRIs, remember that these numbers are the recommended — not required — safe amounts for people in each age and gender group. Look for more information on nutrient recommendations in the nutrition chapters.

Protein: the essential body-builder

Power up and heal with protein

Protein is one nutrient your body absolutely needs to function. It's in every cell in your body, and no other nutrient plays as many different roles in keeping you alive and healthy. Protein's most important job is to build and repair tissue, but it also:

- provides the enzymes and hormones you need for metabolism, digestion, and other critical processes.
- maintains your body's fluid balance.
- carries nutrients throughout your body.
- helps your immune system fight infection and your blood clot properly.

Your body creates this amazing nutrient from 20 building blocks called amino acids. Nine of these are essential amino acids, which means you must get them from food. The others are nonessential. You still need them, but your body can make them, so you don't have to get them from other sources. Your body can't store protein like it does fat and carbohydrates, so you need a new supply of amino acids every day.

What's the best way to get them? Animal-based products like beef, poultry, fish, milk, cheese, and eggs are the top sources because they contain all the essential amino acids. They are known as complete, or high-quality, proteins. Some crops, like soybeans and quinoa, are complete proteins, but most plants are incomplete because they don't have all the amino acids. Nuts, seeds, beans, grains, and vegetables are examples of incomplete proteins.

If plant foods are the mainstay of your diet, you don't have to worry. Simply combine incomplete proteins to get the full range of amino acids your body needs. Rice and beans is a typical combination that does the job. Or take a cue from your childhood, and eat a peanut butter sandwich. You don't have to eat the complementary proteins in the same meal — just make sure it's the same day.

Because protein is such a critical nutrient, you need to make sure you get enough each day. The Recommended Dietary Allowance (RDA) is 46 grams (g) for adult women and 56 g for men. But your body needs to replace protein tissue every day, so larger people actually have a higher protein need than those who weigh less. To figure out what's right for you, multiply 0.36 grams for each pound of body weight. If you weigh 140 pounds, you'll find you need 50 g of protein to meet your daily requirements.

But don't overdo it. An overload of protein can strain your liver and kidneys and make it more difficult for your body to absorb other nutrients. Plus eating lots of meat can overload your body with saturated fat and cholesterol. A 9-ounce T-bone steak, for example, contains a whopping 62 g of protein, 20 g of saturated fat, and 168 milligrams of cholesterol. Look for healthy protein choices like low-fat milk and yogurt or fat-free cheese.

Experts recommend you include protein-rich foods at each meal to reap the most benefit. To get a balanced supply throughout the day, choose foods like these:

- 1 cup oatmeal 6 g
- 8 oz Greek yogurt 17 g
- 3 oz beef or poultry 25 g
- 1 cup edamame 17 g
- 1 oz almonds 6 g
- 1 cup low-fat milk 8 g
- 1 egg 6 g
- 1 cup quinoa 8 g
- half cup black beans 7 g
- 1 oz pumpkin seeds 5 g

CAUTION

Don't get burned by your beef

In summer, there's nothing like the smell of a delicious steak on a charcoal grill. But don't let it get too fired up. Flames and high temperatures can brand your foods with cancer-causing agents called heterocyclic amines (HCAs) and polycyclic aromatic hydrocarbons (PAHs). Any high-temperature cooking, including pan frying and broiling, can put you at risk. To lower the likelihood of creating HCAs and PAHs:

- cook meat medium-rare or medium rather than well-done.
- partially cook meat in the microwave before throwing it on the grill.
- add barbecue sauce to your meat at the end of grilling to lessen charring.
- marinate meat in an oil-free mixture using an acid like vinegar or lemon juice.
- mix chopped cherries into your ground beef for flavor as well as cancer protection.
- skip the grill and use a slower, moister method, like stewing or braising.

Preserve your pizzazz with protein

You can stay active no matter what your age, plus help your body ward off disease, just by getting the right amount of protein each day. This simple addition to your diet plan may be just what your body needs.

Research shows that up to 24 percent of older women are protein deficient because they're eating fewer protein-rich foods. To make matters worse, the older you get, the harder it is for your body to absorb and process protein. That means it's struggling to build and maintain your cells and tissues without the critical building blocks it needs. Add more protein to your diet, and you'll give your body a fighting chance. Here are some ways it can help.

Maintains muscle strength. You naturally lose muscle mass as you age, but losing muscle strength and function leads to a serious condition known as sarcopenia. Physical activity, particularly strength training, is the best way to prevent this condition. But research also suggests older adults can combat muscle decline by eating more protein. A seven-year study of 5,000 postmenopausal women found that those who included more protein in their diets functioned better physically than those who got the fewest calories from protein.

Supports your heart. Remember, your heart is a muscle, and protein helps build muscle. But you need to get the right kind of protein to strengthen your heart and fight off disease. Research shows that eating protein-rich foods like nuts, fish, poultry and low-fat dairy significantly lowers your risk of heart disease compared with eating red meat, processed meats, and high-fat dairy.

Battles osteoporosis. Experts used to think excess protein hurt bone density by leaching out calcium. Instead, recent research suggests protein may work with calcium to prevent bone loss. In one study, scientists found that older women's bones may benefit from more protein, especially if their calcium levels are low. Another study showed that supplementing with the amino acids phenylalanine, tyrosine, and tryptophan helped increase bone mass in older animals.

Balances blood sugar levels. Adding protein to your morning meal could be just the thing to even out your glucose levels and lower your risk of developing diabetes. And if you have type 2 diabetes, studies show that including protein and healthy fat in a hearty breakfast may help you control blood sugar as well as hunger.

Although the RDA for adult women is 46 grams, don't be afraid to eat more. New research from Purdue University suggests older women would benefit from eating 29 percent more protein than recommended daily, or about 59 grams.

"Our data suggests that the current dietary protein requirement estimate may be too low and reinforces that more research is needed to identify accurate protein amounts for older adults," says nutrition science professor Wayne W. Campbell, an expert on dietary protein and human health.

"These findings, along with previous research, indicate that consuming amounts of protein moderately above the current RDA may be helpful."

How safe is soy?

Soy is a complete protein so it's often the food of choice for vegetarians who want to meet their protein needs. It was hailed as a wonder food for many years, with supporters claiming it lowers your risk of breast cancer and also helps your heart, bones, and menopausal symptoms.

Researchers have credited estrogen-like compounds called isoflavones for soy's apparent disease-fighting properties.

But soy may be a proverbial wolf in sheep's clothing. Negative research shows it may impact brain function and memory and possibly contribute to Alzheimer's disease. Other research says it may affect your thyroid and prevent your body from absorbing vital nutrients like iron and zinc.

If you want to include soy in your diet, eating a moderate amount of whole soy foods like soybeans, soy milk, tofu, tempeh, and miso are the best options.

Stay away from isolated and refined forms like soy isolates, soy concentrates, hydrolyzed and textured soy protein, and textured vegetable protein. You'll find these in many processed foods but also in unexpected sources like canned tuna, breads, fast-food burgers, and ice cream.

Quality carbs: put more pep in your step

Rev up your body with nature's energizers

Does the word carbohydrate conjure up pictures of apples, spinach, yogurt, or candy? Probably not. Most people don't realize these foods all contain carbohydrates. And just like the more well-known carbs in bread and pasta, they're your body's major source of energy. Cut out the carbs, and your body will suffer.

Carbohydrates get a bad rap because many people believe high-carb foods make you gain weight. But these super nutrients have important jobs like fueling your brain and central nervous system, keeping your digestive system regular, and providing the energy you need to keep your body moving. Jump on the low-carb bandwagon long enough, and you may end up feeling weak, dizzy, and constipated.

Even worse, when your body can't find carbohydrates for fuel, it will steal protein from your muscles for energy instead. When protein is broken down to make the sugar glucose, it can no longer be used to build muscle. That could lead to muscle weakness and kidney stress, along with other serious problems.

Understand the carb-energy connection. A carbohydrate is a compound made up of one or more sugar molecules. It's known as a macronutrient — along with protein and fat — because it's a major nutrient that supplies your body with calories, or energy.

Nutritionists divide carbohydrates into two groups — simple and complex — based on the number of molecules they have. You're probably familiar with some simple sugars like glucose, fructose, sucrose, and lactose. Starch and fiber are examples of complex carbohydrates.

Your body breaks down all carbohydrates into simple sugars, which the bloodstream absorbs. As your blood sugar levels rise, your pancreas releases a hormone called insulin to move the sugar from your blood into the cells, where it's used for energy.

The type of food you eat determines how quickly your blood sugar rises. For instance, when you bite into a food loaded with simple sugars like an apple or candy bar, your blood absorbs the sugars quickly, and your sugar levels spike. This sudden rise delivers a brief — but not lasting — burst of energy.

Plus, you'll feel hungry again fairly soon. Complex carbs make your blood sugar rise slowly and steadily and deliver long-lasting fuel. That's because your body digests them before absorbing them into your bloodstream. Complex carbs also satisfy your hunger longer.

Your body needs both types of energy for exercise. So here's a tip — before going for a walk, get a quick energy boost by drinking a cup of juice or eating a piece of toast with jelly. During a workout, munch on a handful of pretzels to keep going. Afterwards, you need a light meal to restock your muscles with carbs. Try a granola bar or a bowl of cereal.

Know your daily needs. Eating the right amount of carbohydrates every day is as important as brushing your teeth. To meet your needs based on the Dietary Reference Intakes (DRI), try to get 45 to 65 percent of your calories from carbohydrates.

That means if you eat around 2,000 calories a day, 900 to 1,300 of those calories should come from carbs. Or check packages for grams, and aim for 225 to 325 per day. Here's what a typical day might look like.

Carbohydrate foods	Grams	Calories
1 cup oatmeal	56	307
1 cup reduced-fat milk	12	122
2 slices whole wheat toast	26	152
1 cup low-fat fruit yogurt	47	250
1 apple	25	95
1 banana	27	105
1 sweet potato	24	105
1/2 cup chocolate ice cream	19	143
Total	236	1,279

Pick carbs packed with nutrients. Bite into a plump peach, and you'll taste the sweetness of fructose. Nibble on a piece of chocolate, and your mouth will melt with the sugary sensation of sucrose. Both are delicious, but one gives you a burst of nutrition, and the other, mostly empty calories.

- Use the glycemic index (GI) — a chart that classifies foods depending on how quickly or slowly they raise your blood sugar. If you struggle with diabetes, the GI can help you make smart choices. For more about the glycemic index, see Can glycemic index help control blood sugar? in the *Diabetes: outwit a deadly diagnosis* chapter.

- Limit cakes and cookies that are full of sucrose or other added sugars. They provide few, if any, nutrients. An apple or banana loaded with natural fructose also delivers essential vitamins and minerals — a healthier choice.

- Choose whole grains over refined ones, and eat beans, peas, brown or wild rice, nuts and seeds, and vegetables with lots of fiber like broccoli and zucchini.

Without question, your body needs carbohydrates, so don't get swayed by popular opinion and cut these valuable nutrients out of your diet. Just make a point of eating nutrient-rich carbs. You'll reap tremendous health benefits, including the energy your brain and body need to get through each day.

Quick way to identify a healthy carb

It's a classic case of good vs. evil. In one corner, you have carbs that can battle depression, anxiety, and prostate cancer. In the other, you have carbs that can lead to weight gain, diabetes, and heart disease. So how do you know which is which?

Some carbs, like fruits, vegetables, and whole grains, deliver an abundance of fiber and the nutrients your body needs for healthy living. They're also rich in important phytonutrients — plant chemicals that promote good health.

Others offer few to no nutrients. Manufacturers enrich some of these carbs with vitamins and minerals, but they can still contain too much fat, added sugar and salt, and preservatives.

Your best bet is to read food labels and apply this simple formula created to help identify healthy whole-grain foods. Researchers at Harvard University have tested and endorsed it, but you don't have to be a math whiz to use it.

Step 1 — Read a nutrition label and look for the amount of dietary fiber and total number of carbohydrates.

Step 2 — Multiply the fiber by 10.

Step 3 — If the number is equal to or greater than the total carbs, then stock up — you've picked a nutrient-rich carb.

You can apply this formula to any food to determine if it's a "good" carb. For example, a package of dried fruits and nuts — almonds, raisins, cherries, cranberries, and pistachios — contains 16 grams of total carbs and 2 grams of fiber.

- 10 times 2 equals 20.
- 20 is higher than 16.
- The snack is a high-quality carb.

Don't be fooled by sneaky bread labels

No matter how you slice it, life without bread is no life at all. But how do you know which breads are best for you? The answer is easy — whole grains.

Unfortunately, manufacturers like to put health claims like "all natural" and "multigrain" on bread bags. These claims can deceive you if you don't know what to look for.

Here's how to know which breads contain whole grains, and which ones don't.

- Make sure the nutrition label says 100-percent whole-wheat or 100-percent whole grain as the first ingredient.
- Ignore packages with words like wheat, multigrain, seven-grain, and cracked wheat. Many manufacturers use these words to imply their breads are made with whole grains, but they're not.
- Look for the 100-percent whole-grain stamp. This seal provided by the Whole Grains Council, a nonprofit that promotes the health benefits of whole grains, ensures you are buying a legit loaf of whole-grain bread.
- Learn to spot whole grains such as barley, buckwheat, millet, quinoa, whole oats, whole rye, and whole-wheat.
- Put anything that says "unbleached" or "enriched" wheat flour back on the shelf. That's just another way of saying white flour.

- Don't buy a loaf of bread just because it's brown. The color doesn't mean it's whole-wheat.
- Scan the list of ingredients for salt. Since most loaves of bread contain about one teaspoon of salt, and ingredients are listed in descending order by amount, any grain listed after salt would be insignificant.

Now it's time to test your knowledge. Can you pick out the healthiest bread from the two lists below?

Multigrain	Whole-wheat
INGREDIENTS: Unbleached Enriched Wheat Flour, Water, Wheat Gluten, Cellulose, Yeast, Soybean Oil, Honey, **Salt**, Barley, Natural Flavor Preservatives, Monocalcium Phosphate, Millet, Corn, Oats, Soybean Flour, Brown Rice, Flaxseed.	INGREDIENTS: 100% Whole-Grain Whole-Wheat Flour, Water, Oat Fiber, Wheat Gluten, Yeast, Brown Sugar, Contains 2% Or Less Of The Following: **Salt**, Dough Conditioners, Fumaric Acid, Yeast Nutrients, Flaxseed, Wheat Starch, Calcium Propionate, Potassium Sorbate, Natamycin And Gamma Cyclodextrin, Soy Lecithin.

If you picked the whole-wheat bread, give yourself an A+. This loaf contains 100-percent whole-wheat. The multigrain bread lists unbleached enriched wheat flour as its first ingredient. This is not a whole grain. And the label mentions barley, millet, corn, oats, and brown rice after salt, so this bread includes minimal amounts of those grains.

Latest scoop on controversial sweetener

Gulp down a sugary soda, and your taste buds explode with the sweetness of high-fructose corn syrup (HFCS). Many critics believe HFCS is harmful — more harmful than other added sugars. But others say it's no better or worse than any other sugar.

This popular sweetener is a combination of two simple sugars — fructose and glucose. Because HFCS tastes sweeter than regular sugar, manufacturers can use less, which saves them money. You'll find HFCS in everything from soda to pancake syrup. Scientists spend a lot of time studying HFCS, and what they're learning may surprise you.

- Too much high-fructose corn syrup can lead to weight gain and more belly fat, Princeton University researchers found during an animal study. That's a concern because those conditions can trigger heart disease and diabetes.
- More people suffer from type 2 diabetes in countries that use a lot of HFCS than countries that don't. Researchers from the University of Southern California, after comparing data from 43 countries, made this interesting discovery.
- On the other hand, a team of researchers recently debunked the theory that large amounts of high-fructose corn syrup contributes to nonalcoholic fatty liver disease. After reviewing studies, they found no link between the two, according to their article published in the *American Journal of Clinical Nutrition.*

While research over high-fructose corn syrup continues, many experts say the real issue is not the added sugar itself — it's people's obsession with all added sugars. They just can't get enough. And that in itself causes problems. For example, people who drink sodas don't feel as full as people who get the same number of calories from food so they tend to eat just as much as if they hadn't guzzled a soft drink, says a Harvard School of Public Health study. It's not necessarily the HFCS — it's that soft drinks don't fill you up like other carbs. This tendency to overeat is a major problem, says Dr. John Sievenpiper, a researcher at St. Michael's Hospital in Toronto.

"The debate over the role of fructose in obesity, fatty liver, and other metabolic diseases has distracted us from the issue of overconsumption," he says. "Our data should serve to remind people that the excess calories, whether they are from fructose or other sources, are the issue."

The message is clear — no matter what type of added sugar you are talking about, cut back.

Short-circuit sugar cravings

Most Americans get about 30 teaspoons of added sugar every day. That's a whopping 228 cups a year. But extra pounds aren't the only problem with added sugar. Your chances of dying from heart disease go way up when you guzzle too much of the sweet stuff. In fact, the risk jumped 38 percent for people in a recent study who got 17 to 21 percent of their calories from added sugar compared to those who got just 8 percent. Drink three cans of regular soda, and you'll reach that upper limit.

Other studies show added sugar may raise blood pressure, triglyceride levels, and LDL cholesterol, and contribute to inflammation — all key factors in heart disease. Bitter news if you have a sweet tooth. Thankfully, you don't have to give up sweet treats completely to maintain good health. You just need to know your limits. Keep these suggestions in mind the next time you crave something sweet.

Know how low you should go. No one likes to count grams and calories — especially for sweets. But if you want to live healthy, you need to know how much sugar is too much. Look at the table below with recommendations from the *Dietary Guidelines for Americans.* If you eat this many calories a day, don't eat or drink more than this much added sugar.

To put things in perspective, think about this. A 12-ounce can of soda contains around 38 grams of sugar. That's more than 8 teaspoons, too much sugar for one day if you eat around 2,000 calories.

1,600 calories	4 teaspoons or about 16 grams
1,800 calories	5 teaspoons or about 20 grams
2,000 to 2,200 calories	8 teaspoons or about 32 grams
2,400 calories	10 teaspoons or 40 grams

Solve the secret to sugar names. Added sugars parade across food labels with sneaky names. Here's an easy way to find them. If a word ends in -ose like maltose and sucrose, it's an added sugar. Other added sugars end with the words "syrup" like corn syrup or "concentrate" as in fruit juice concentrate. But remember, new food labels will show the amount of added sugars in grams. To see a revised nutrition panel, turn to *New food label cuts the confusion* earlier in Step 2.

Sweet ways to swap out sugar. As you cut back on sugar, you may need a few ideas to get you through the day. Here's a list to get you started.

- Sweeten bland foods like oatmeal with spices like cloves, nutmeg, cinnamon, or allspice.
- Slash the amount of sugar you use in recipes by up to a third without changing the taste. Or swap out sugar with almond, lemon, orange, or vanilla extract.
- Dip a banana or berries in chocolate for a sweet but nutritious treat.
- Eat regular meals that combine protein, whole grains, fruits, and vegetables throughout your day. This will keep your blood sugar stable and cut out cravings for sweets.

Fiber: a nutritional big shot

Slash fat and inches with hearty grains

What's the number one food for reducing your cholesterol? Here's a hint — its side effect is a slimmer waist. If you guessed oats, you guessed right.

Oats contain a sensational soluble fiber called beta-glucan. Experts say beta-glucan can flush out your arteries, lowering your cholesterol and battling heart disease.

Scientists think one way fiber lowers cholesterol is by binding with bile acids. The liver makes bile acids from cholesterol to help with digestion. When fiber ferries these acids out of your system, your liver grabs cholesterol from your bloodstream to make more bile. The result is less cholesterol floating around wreaking havoc in your arteries.

If you want a change from oats, try barley, another grain rich in beta-glucan. Just a quarter cup of uncooked pearl barley daily can dissolve cholesterol and open up arteries. That's about a cup of cooked barley with its 3 grams of beta-glucan. New research published in the *European Journal of Clinical Nutrition* suggests that eating 3 grams of barley beta-glucan every day lowers cholesterol.

Look in the rice or dried beans section of your favorite supermarket for this top-notch heart healer. Add barley to soups, pasta dishes, and hot cereals for this heart-healthy grain. Or try hulled barley, which has the most fiber of any whole grain.

Beta-glucan boasts one other fabulous benefit — it fills you up without filling you out, says a study published in the *Journal of the American Dietetic Association*. Researchers asked 500 overweight and obese adults to eat 500 less calories a day. Half the group ate two servings of oat cereal daily, and the other half ate a low-fiber breakfast with the same amount of calories. After just four weeks, the group that ate oat cereal lost more inches and had lower cholesterol levels than the other group.

And it's not just oats. Barley expands in your stomach, leaving you feeling fuller for longer. In fact, a review published by the Department of Agriculture shows that eating whole grains, in general, lowers your body fat, trims your waist, and reduces your risk for gaining weight.

So make sure you stock up on oats and barley, fill up on beta-glucan, and start reaping the benefits.

CAUTION

Supplement warning you should not ignore

Taking fiber supplements, including the herb psyllium, could interfere with the absorption of medications you take and minerals you need. Fiber sweeps them through your digestive system without giving them time to get fully absorbed.

- Medications — If you take drugs for your heart, cholesterol, or diabetes, experts suggest taking fiber supplements two to three hours before or after you take your medications. These include popular prescriptions like Crestor, Plavix, and Lipitor.
- Minerals — Your body needs iron, zinc, calcium, and magnesium for good health. But eating too much fiber can bind with these minerals and flush them out of your body before you can absorb them. Stick to eating the recommended daily allowance — 25 grams a day for women and 38 grams a day for men — and fiber shouldn't be a problem.

5 reasons to give fiber a high-five

You want your digestive system to run as smoothly as a well-oiled machine. Only fiber can do that, and so much more. It's the secret weapon that supercharges your digestive health.

Your body cannot digest fiber. This gives it a chance to slide through your digestive tract, slowing down or speeding up digestion. The speed of digestion depends on which type of fiber you're eating — soluble or insoluble.

Soluble fiber absorbs water like a sponge, but turns into a gel as it slowly glides through your gut. Beans, nuts, berries, and oatmeal pack powerful amounts of soluble fiber.

Insoluble fiber bulks up and softens your stool and helps it sail through your intestines. When you eat barley, brown rice, whole-grain cereals, and some fruits and vegetables with their skins, you're getting insoluble fiber.

Most fruits and vegetables deliver a one-two punch, providing both kinds of fiber. For instance, a pear has over 2 grams of soluble fiber and almost 4 grams of insoluble fiber. And a half cup of sweet potato boasts almost 2 grams of soluble fiber and over 2 grams of insoluble.

Eating both types of fiber daily fights all sorts of digestive distress. Here's a look at what sensational fiber can do for you.

Conquers constipation. Everyone's bowel habits are different, but many doctors say you're constipated if you go to the bathroom less than three times a week. And while constipation can mean you're not drinking enough water or getting enough exercise, it could just mean you're not getting enough fiber. Try drinking plenty of water and eating insoluble fiber like fruits, veggies, or whole grains.

Defeats diarrhea. Bacteria, parasites, viruses, even some medications can keep you running to the bathroom. To treat mild to moderate cases, try soluble fiber like oatmeal, bananas, and mashed potatoes. These foods will soak up water from your intestines and firm up your stool.

Guards against gallstones. Many people go through life with gallstones and don't know it. But those who do, suffer severe pain, fever, chills, and vomiting. Gallstones form when bile salts containing cholesterol crystallize. Their sizes range from a grain of sand to a golf ball. These stones can block the passage between your gallbladder and your liver.

Soluble fiber soaks up bile salts and flushes them out of your system. Insoluble fiber carries food through your gut quickly, so bile doesn't have time to form stones in your gallbladder.

Soothes irritable bowel syndrome. If you suffer from frequent bouts of diarrhea and constipation, plus bloating, nausea, and headaches, you may have irritable bowel syndrome (IBS). No one really knows why people develop IBS, but some doctors believe stress or foods that produce gas play a role. Relieve symptoms with foods high in soluble fiber — apples, strawberries, oats, nuts, and seeds. Stay away from high-fiber wheat bran. It could make IBS worse.

Calms ulcers. Although the bacterium *H. pylori* causes most ulcers, you're also at risk if you take nonsteroidal anti-inflammatory drugs (NSAIDs), like ibuprofen and aspirin, for arthritis. These painful sores usually affect the stomach or the first part of your small intestine. Some studies show eating high-fiber foods lowers your risk of getting ulcers. Soluble fibers seem to lessen the amount of stomach acid your body makes, which can help ulcers heal.

If you're not used to eating a lot of fiber, add it gradually and drink plenty of liquids. Too much fiber can make you feel gassy, crampy, and bloated. Follow the *Dietary Guidelines for Americans*, which recommends a daily total of 25 grams for women and 38 grams for men.

6 surprisingly tasty sources of fiber

If you think fiber tastes like cardboard, you're in for a surprise. These treats will tickle your taste buds while serving up a healthy dose of fiber.

- Grapefruit — Skip the juice and go straight for the fruit. This citrus sweetheart packs up fiber in a gel-like substance called pectin.
- Olives — Toss these in a salad or pasta dish for a savory source of fiber.
- Artichoke hearts — Sauté in a little bit of olive oil with garlic, and add to a casserole to boost fiber without a lot of calories.
- Hazelnuts — Go nuts over this fabulous source of fiber. Half a cup serves up about 6 grams. Toss them into a fruit salad for a crunchy treat.
- Dark chocolate — Let a 1.4-ounce serving melt in your mouth, and you'll enjoy a jumbo serving of fiber — about 3 to 6 grams.
- Raspberries — Enjoy a cup of raspberries for a whopping 8 grams of fiber. They taste great over plain yogurt or a bowl of whole-grain cereal.

An amazing cancer fighter everyone needs

It's no surprise fiber can help prevent colon and stomach cancers. After all, it acts like a broom, sweeping away toxins from your digestive system. But did you know getting your daily fill of fiber could fight off a number of other cancers?

Prostate. Roughly 15 men out of every 100 will get prostate cancer at some point during their lifetime. Fortunately, that number is dropping, and fiber could be the reason. Researchers at the University of Sorbonne in Paris studied more than 3,000 men for over 12 years. They found that the more insoluble fiber the men ate the lower their risk of prostate cancer. The fiber from legumes like peas, beans, lentils, and peanuts seems to work best. Other studies show that eating high-fiber foods may keep prostate cancer cells from multiplying.

Kidney. You don't hear much about kidney cancer because only a tiny number of Americans get it — about 15 out of 100,000. Even so, eating fiber-rich foods like fruits, vegetables, and whole grains might help keep it away. Experts think fiber prevents cancer-causing toxins from reaching your kidneys.

Breast. No woman wants to hear the words, "You have breast cancer." But every year well over 200,000 American woman do. Studies show that eating soluble fiber lowers the risk of breast cancer because it helps your body excrete estrogen.

Researchers agree they need to do more research. In the meantime, a high-fiber, plant-based diet promotes good health. So why not start eating more fiber now?

Surprising way to boost helpful gut bugs

Your gut is like a Star Wars convention, playing host to trillions of alien bugs. These bugs, also known as good bacteria or probiotics, help digest food, battle harmful bacteria, and boost your immune system — all great reasons to keep them around. That's where fiber comes in.

Probiotics need something to eat, and they love to feast on fiber. Experts call fiber "prebiotic" because they help your probiotics grow and thrive. That keeps you and your gut healthy.

So the next time you eat a bowl of bean soup or a piece of whole-wheat toast, enjoy the probiotic party going on in your belly.

Fats: the ones to pick, the ones to pitch

Get the skinny on fabulous fats

Fat is not just the jiggly stuff around your belly and thighs. It's a nutrient every person needs to stay healthy. Surprised? Most people are, considering "fat" is like a four-letter word today. But as you learn more about nutrition, you'll realize fat is something you can't live without.

Scientists divide fats into three categories — body fat, cholesterol, and dietary fats. They're all related, but certainly not the same.

You need a certain amount of good dietary fats to stay healthy. These fats pour on the benefits without packing on inches or wreaking havoc in your arteries. In fact, the good fats found in nuts, plants, and fish deliver a slew of benefits to your body.

- When you exercise, you use carbs for energy for the first 20 minutes. But then it's the calories from fat that give you the energy you need to keep going.
- Your body can't absorb vitamins A, D, E, and K without fat. That's why they're called fat-soluble vitamins.
- Fats make foods flavorful and help you feel full.
- Your fat cells need fats to insulate your body and keep you warm.

- Your hair and skin need fats to stay healthy.

But beware — fats are not created equal. Saturated fats can trigger life-threatening heart disease and the blood clotting associated with heart attacks.

Think butter, shortening, and the white marbled fat in meat — all of these are solid at room temperature. And they're loaded with saturated fat. Limit these by eating no more than 10 percent or 22 grams of saturated fat a day based on a 2,000-calorie diet.

On the other hand, unsaturated fats keep you healthy and battle disease. You find these liquid fats in nuts, fish, and vegetable oils like olive, canola, and safflower. These fats are broken down into two groups — monounsaturated (MUFA) and polyunsaturated (PUFA). You need both for optimal health.

Pump up the PUFAs. You've probably heard of omega-3 fatty acids, the polyunsaturated fats you get from fish like salmon, tuna, and halibut. But you probably don't know your body can't make omega-3. So you need to find ways to get it into your diet. Research shows this fat helps prevent cancer and heart disease, reduces inflammation, and keeps your mind and memory sharp.

A distant cousin to omega-3 is omega-6 fatty acid. They're similar in that your body can't make omega-6 either, so you have to get it from food. Studies show omega-6 promotes brain function, lowers blood pressure, and reduces your risk of diabetes.

The key to getting the greatest health benefits from these two fatty acids is balance. Omega-3 seems to reduce inflammation, while some omega-6 fatty acids promote it. The ideal ratio of omega-6 to omega-3 is 4 to 1, but the typical American diet is closer to 20 to 1.

Eating more fish, fresh fruits and vegetables, whole grains, garlic, and olive oil — and less meat — can help you achieve a healthy balance. These food choices are typical of the Mediterranean Diet.

To read more about this heart-healthy diet, see the related story in the *Inflammation: stamp out the source of disease* chapter.

Maximize the MUFAs. This type of fat is found in a variety of foods and oils, including nuts like macadamias and hazelnuts, and oils like olive and safflower. Studies show eating foods rich in MUFA may control insulin and blood sugar levels, which is especially helpful for people with type 2 diabetes.

Boost your good fats. Choose fats wisely to reap the benefits. Experts recommend you get 20 percent to 35 percent of your daily total calories from fats, primarily unsaturated fats. Here's a list of ideas to get you started.

- Bake, grill, broil, or steam foods instead of frying.
- Trade meat for seafood like salmon or mackerel twice a week. Stick with a 4-ounce serving.
- Pick fat-free or low-fat cheese, milk, and ice cream over those loaded with fat.
- Use olive oil to make marinades and salad dressings, and to sauté vegetables.
- Add flavor to your foods with herbs, lemon juice, salsa, vinegar, or broth-based sauces.
- Steer clear of solid fats like lard and butter. Go with olive or canola oil, or a margarine that lists liquid vegetable oil as its first ingredient.
- Trim the skin from chicken and excess fat from steaks before cooking.
- Look for the number of fat grams on Nutrition Facts labels when you shop for groceries.

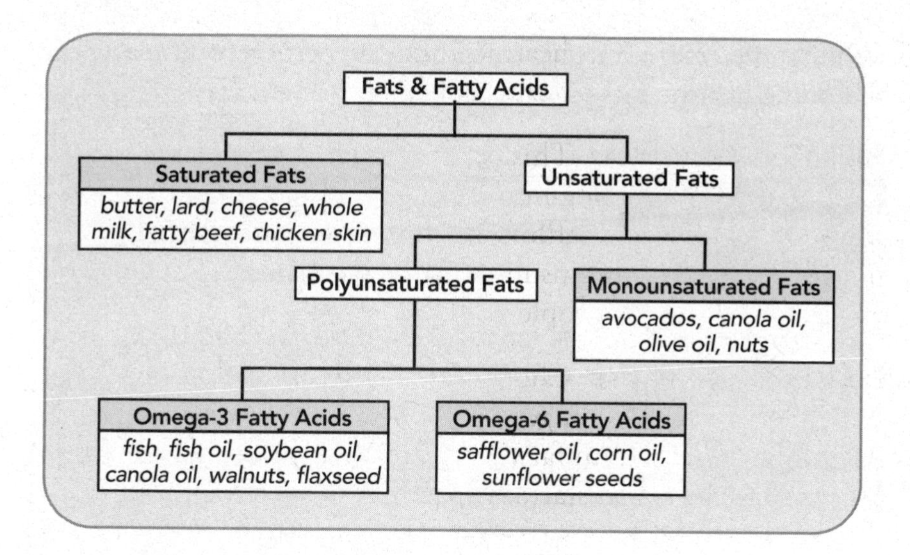

Does low-fat dieting harm your heart?

Low-fat diets can create chaos in your body, including weight gain. Before you jump on the low-fat bandwagon, get the latest facts.

- Food manufacturers pour added sugar into low-fat foods to make them taste better. The label may say low-fat, but the calories can be through the roof. What's more, these foods raise your blood triglycerides and lower your good HDL cholesterol — a dangerous combo for your heart.

- Low-fat diets exclude foods like nuts, seeds, fish, and vegetable oils, which are bursting with nutrients. So you don't get the vitamins, minerals, and phytochemicals you need for a healthy heart.

- Research shows low-fat diets may lower bad cholesterol, but not the risk of dying from heart disease.

- Several studies from the Women's Health Initiative suggest that older women eating low-fat diets did not lower their risk for stroke, heart disease, breast cancer, or colon cancer. The study followed post-menopausal women for over eight years.

While more research needs to be done, experts recommend you add some healthy fats to your daily diet.

Trans fat alert: a cholesterol double whammy

Trans fats spell trouble for you. They raise your bad LDL cholesterol and lower your good HDL cholesterol, increasing your risk of heart disease. That's why the Food and Drug Administration wants to ban them.

Manufacturers take polyunsaturated oils and turn them into trans fats using a process called hydrogenation. This makes the oils solid and more stable, helping foods stay fresher longer.

Many health experts believe lowering the amount of trans fats in the American diet could prevent 20,000 heart attacks and 7,000 deaths from heart disease a year. But many bakers disagree. They believe trans fats in trace amounts are not harmful and are a critical ingredient in many baked goods.

As the debate continues, you can protect your health by reading food labels. Avoid packages with the words "trans fat" or "partially hydrogenated oils."

The mega benefits of omega-3s

I'll bet you didn't know you don't need to take pain pills — tuna can ease arthritis. Why? Because it's loaded with omega-3 fatty acids, the nutrient that works as well as medicine for relieving your arthritis pain.

Your body can't make omega-3s, but you can get this amazing nutrient from salmon and other fish, which are rich in two omega-3 fatty acids — docosahexaenoic acid (DHA) and eicosapentaenoic acid (EPA). These two fatty acids battle inflammation. And inflammation, scientists say, may be the root of many chronic conditions like high blood pressure, cancer, depression, diabetes, and arthritis.

Experts believe omega-3s work by blocking two of your body's chemicals — cytokines and prostaglandins — that trigger inflammation. They also pump up your body's anti-inflammatory chemicals called resolvins. This one-two punch can knock out all sorts of health problems.

Soothe achy joints. Imagine feeling sweet pain relief without popping a pill. That's what omega-3s can do for people with arthritis. Several studies show that omega-3s from fish can ease morning stiffness and lessen the need for nonsteroidal anti-inflammatory drugs (NSAIDs). This is great news for people with chronic pain because NSAIDs can cause stomach bleeding, as well as heart and kidney problems.

Preserve your memories. You never want to forget meaningful events. But Alzheimer's can rob you of those memories. Thankfully, researchers at Columbia University found that eating fish can fend off dementia in people with mild memory loss. And a study published in the journal *Molecular Nutrition and Food Research* suggests that omega-3 fatty acids may even prevent Alzheimer's.

Keep your ticker ticking. People who eat more than two servings of fish a week show less atherosclerosis in their carotid artery than those who eat little to none. That's what a study in *Nutrition Journal* suggests. And a study published in the *Journal of the American Heart Association* shows eating seafood regularly lowers your risk of heart disease.

Shake off blood sugar problems. Your body uses a hormone called insulin to turn sugar into energy. If your body stops using insulin properly, sugar builds up in your blood. Doctors call this insulin resistance. Many overweight and obese people struggle with this condition, which can lead to type 2 diabetes, high blood pressure, high cholesterol, and heart disease. But omega-3s can help. A study from The Center for Genetics, Nutrition, and Health shows a diet rich in omega-3 fatty acids from seafood curbs the harmful effects of a diet high in sugar.

Now that you know the health benefits of omega-3s, you'll want to go fishing for good sources. Make sure you add the following foods to your shopping list.

- fatty fish, like salmon, mackerel, herring, and tuna
- flaxseed and flaxseed oil
- walnuts
- canola oil

Fish oil supplements: OK or no-way?

Not a fish lover? You're not alone. If you want to add omega-3s to your diet, consider taking supplements — with caution.

Studies show fish oil supplements may reduce the inflammation that can lead to heart disease, diabetes, and memory loss. Combine them with aspirin, and you get a double whammy. Researchers from Brigham and Women's Hospital and Harvard Medical School found that when you take aspirin with fish oil supplements, they work together even better to combat inflammation.

Before you try this combo, talk with your doctor. Fish oil supplements and aspirin can have serious side effects, like thinning your blood. You shouldn't take them if you already take a blood thinner, such as Coumadin (warfarin).

Vitamin-rich foods: what you should be eating now

Revitalize your life with vitamins

In Latin, "vita" means life and "amines" means organic substances. Put the two together and what do you get? Vitamins — organic nutrients that are vital to life.

A healthy diet filled with fruits, vegetables, and whole grains provides all the vitamins you need — 13 in fact. You need these vitamins for your body to grow and digest food. Your nerves also need them to work properly.

Like actors in a movie, each vitamin plays a leading role or supporting role in your body. For example, you need vitamin A to help you see better, especially at night. Vitamin D helps you absorb calcium for healthy bones.

Nutritionists divide vitamins into two groups — fat-soluble and water-soluble.

Vitamins A, D, E, and K are fat-soluble. This simply means your fat cells store them, and your body can hang on to them for weeks, even months. When they're needed, special protein carriers ferry them through your blood.

The B vitamins and vitamin C are water-soluble. Your body absorbs them quickly, and gets rid of any extra in your urine.

It's best to get vitamins from the foods you eat, but people on restrictive diets may need to take supplements. Check with your doctor first.

Read on to learn more about these life-giving nutrients.

5 vitamin myths debunked

Americans shell out a whopping $5 billion in vitamin supplements every year. That's big business for supplement suppliers. And who wouldn't want to take a multivitamin? Their labels make them sound like you can't live without them. But are supplements all they're cracked up to be?

Take, for example, one popular multivitamin that claims it can lower your risk of heart disease. Research shows multivitamins can do no such thing.

To be a savvy health consumer, you need to separate fact from fiction.

Antioxidant vitamins prevent cancer. You've heard this popular myth for decades. But study after study has shown taking antioxidant supplements do nothing to prevent or battle cancer. One alarming piece of research published in the *Annals of Internal Medicine* suggests beta carotene supplements actually raise the risk of lung cancer in people at high risk, like smokers.

A review of 14 trials found the supplements A, C, E, and beta carotene, which were taken to prevent intestinal cancers, actually raised the risk of death. Another study shows vitamin E raises the risk of prostate cancer.

Experts believe it's because antioxidants don't attack cancer cells in the mitochondria part of the cell. That's where cells produce agents that promote tumors. Instead, antioxidants interact with other parts of the cell that don't promote tumors.

Vitamins are "natural" so my doctor doesn't need to know what I take. If you think your vitamin is all-natural, think again. Manufacturers often produce supplements with synthetic additives, then slap the Department of Agriculture's organic seal on the bottles. And it's all legal.

Plus, the Food and Drug Administration doesn't require supplements to undergo rigorous testing like prescription drugs. So the supplement you think you're getting may be spiked with steroids or other ingredients.

Then there's evidence that your supplement can interfere with health conditions, medications, and test results. For instance, vitamin C can botch the outcome of fecal occult blood tests used to detect bleeding in your digestive tract.

Always talk with your doctor about the supplements you take. Buy products with the GMP Certified mark, which stands for "good manufacturing practices." Or look for the USP Verified mark from the nonprofit organization U.S. Pharmacopeia. The supplements with these labels pass tests for strength, quality, purity, and composition.

You can't get too much of a good thing. If 100 percent of the recommended daily allowance is good, then 1,000 percent should be better — right? Wrong!

- A study out of the Karolinska Institute in Sweden found that men who took 1,000 milligrams of vitamin C are twice as likely to develop kidney stones than those who don't take supplements. In the U.S., the Dietary Reference Intake only recommends 90 milligrams of vitamin C for men and 75 milligrams for women, way below the popular dose of 1,000 milligrams sold in drugstores and supermarkets.

- Take a high dose of vitamin A and your whole body will suffer the consequences. The National Institutes of Health says just one dose of more than 40,000 international units can cause severe headaches, nausea, vertigo, blurred vision, muscle aches, and lack of coordination. Taken repeatedly and you're bound to damage your liver.

- Even water-soluble vitamins — the ones your body flushes out what you don't need — can wreak havoc on your body if taken in high doses. Vitamin B6 causes heartburn, nausea, skin irritation, sun sensitivity, and severe nerve damage.

You can eat anything you want as long as you take a multivitamin. You can't fill up on sugary sweets and saturated fats, and expect a multivitamin to undo the damage. And you can't get the fiber found in fruits, veggies, and whole grains, and disease-fighting phytochemicals from a pill. You also need exercise, good sleep, and activities that reduce stress to maintain good health. A supplement can't deliver any of those.

Everyone needs a multivitamin. Experts say don't waste your money. Three studies published in the *Annals of Internal Medicine* show multivitamins offer no health benefits to the average person. If you eat a balanced diet loaded with fruits, vegetables, whole grains, and protein — including dairy, then you're getting all the nutrients you need for a healthy life.

Scientists say the only people who might need a multivitamin are pregnant and nursing moms, people who eat less than 1,200 calories a day or cut out complete food groups like carbs, and those who have trouble digesting or absorbing food. Otherwise, talk with your doctor before starting a vitamin supplement. You probably don't need one. And that's a fact.

3 more reasons to love vitamin C

There's more to "C" than meets the eye. Most people associate this vitamin with the common cold. But new research shows why you need this powerful vitamin as you age.

Safeguards against stroke. An apple a day may keep the doctor away, but an orange a day may save your life. A study from the *American Academy of Neurology* found that people who suffer from hemorrhagic strokes do not get enough vitamin C. This type of stroke occurs when a blood vessel bursts in your brain.

Experts think vitamin C helps by regulating blood pressure and playing an important role in collagen synthesis. Collagen is a protein that helps keep your connective tissue together and your blood vessels from weakening.

Previous studies also show that low vitamin C is linked to heart disease.

Prevents hearing loss. Once upon a time, you may have heard a pin drop. But as you've gotten older, you might have trouble hearing your phone ring or your favorite TV show. Vitamin C can help.

Researchers tested close to 2,000 men and women between the ages of 50 and 80 in a study out of Korea. The study shows that older adults who got more of the super vitamin had better hearing.

Scientists aren't sure why there's a link between low vitamin C and hearing loss. But they do know that older adults tend to eat less foods with vitamin C. A healthy diet loaded with fruits and vegetables should provide plenty.

Keeps your bones strong. Sticks and stones may break your bones. And so will a diet without enough vitamin C. That's why you need more kiwi — a tropical fruit that builds bones and connective tissue.

For years, doctors have known that a lack of vitamin C causes the brittle bones of scurvy. But they didn't know if eating more vitamin C could prevent bone loss.

An animal study from Mount Sinai School of Medicine shows just that. Scientists think vitamin C triggers cells to form bones that protect your skeletal system. It also reduces the risk of fractures.

So go ahead, cut open that kiwi and enjoy the perks of vitamin C.

Latest beta carotene danger

If it wasn't for vitamin A, you wouldn't see well, your immune system wouldn't work right, and your heart, lungs, and kidneys would fail. You don't want anything to get in vitamin A's way. But what if something could?

Research shows beta carotene — the wonderful antioxidant that gives carrots and sweet potatoes their bright, beautiful colors — may block vitamin A from doing its many jobs. Scientists say this happens when you eat excessive amounts of beta carotene. What's interesting is that beta carotene is a "precursor" to vitamin A. That means your body can change beta carotene into vitamin A as needed.

Research suggests the more beta carotene you eat, the more anti-vitamin A molecules there are hanging around. While research continues, researchers aren't suggesting you stop eating foods high in beta carotene, but you might want to avoid excessive amounts.

Breathe easy with this 'E'ssential vitamin

You take over 670 million breaths by the time you reach the age of 80. But what if you have asthma or some other lung condition? Every breath you take is a struggle. It doesn't have to be. Thanks to vitamin E, your lungs can get a second wind.

Vitamin E is a fat-soluble nutrient made up of eight related substances. Experts say two of these — alpha-tocopherol and gamma-tocopherol — can affect your breathing.

Eat corn, soybean, or canola oil and you're getting gamma-tocopherol. This form of vitamin E makes your lungs work harder, suggests a Northwestern University study. Scientists say when gamma-tocopherol binds with a special protein called kinase C-alpha, it increases inflammation in your lungs.

But when this protein binds with alpha-tocopherol, inflammation clears up. You can find alpha-tocopherol in oils like olive, almond, sunflower, and wheat germ, plus nuts, seeds, and leafy green vegetables.

Researchers also noted that countries with low rates of asthma eat a lot more olive and sunflower oils than in America. The rate of asthma in the U.S. has climbed over the past 40 years, and coincides with higher use of corn, soybean, and canola oils.

Surprising way to grow hair

Can a common vitamin re-grow thinning hair? This study suggests it.

Volunteers with significant hair loss took a supplement of tocotrienol — a form of vitamin E — for eight months during this trial from the University of Science Malaysia. All of the volunteers had experienced hair loss for two to five years prior to the study. Those who took 100 milligrams of tocotrienol daily grew more hair than those who took a placebo.

More research needs to be done, so talk with your doctor before taking a vitamin E supplement for hair loss.

Sunshine vitamin shields against arthritis

Don't suffer needlessly from stiffness, pain, and swelling. Prevent arthritis with the vitamin most Americans don't get enough of — vitamin D.

Research shows this valuable vitamin can help keep rheumatoid arthritis (RA) at bay. RA is an autoimmune disease in which your immune system attacks your body's tissues, causing joint pain and swelling mostly in the wrist and fingers.

If you already suffer from RA's achy joints, vitamin D might also slow the disease's progression. Experts believe vitamin D lowers the proteins in your body that set off inflammation.

During the 11-year Iowa Women's Health Study, 152 out of almost 30,000 women developed rheumatoid arthritis. Scientists found that older women who got the most vitamin D, from food or supplements, did not develop RA like women low in vitamin D. In fact, women who got less than 200 international units (IU) each day were 33 percent more likely to develop RA than those who got more.

Another study published in the *British Medical Journal* shows that exposure to ultraviolet B sunlight lowers the risk of rheumatoid arthritis in women between ages 30 and 55. Researchers believe it's the skin's production of vitamin D that fends off the onset of this debilitating condition.

But osteoarthritis (OA) is a different story. OA develops as you age, and often affects your hands, knees, hips, and spine. Studies show that vitamin D doesn't make much difference in people with OA, though more research needs to be done.

Still, your body needs vitamin D to absorb calcium, and calcium is crucial for healthy bones. But a report published in the *Archives of Internal Medicine* suggests up to 75 percent of Americans don't get enough vitamin D.

Boost your intake by spending 10 to 15 minutes in the sun a few times a week and drinking skim or low-fat milk. Or ask your doctor about taking a daily vitamin D supplement.

Tasty ways to preserve vitamins

Raw is better than cooked in many cases. But getting fruits and vegetables from farm to table without losing vitamins and other nutrients is nearly impossible. Here's how you can protect nutrients when you buy and cook produce.

Pick farm fresh. Not everyone has a farm stand near home. But if you do, locally grown produce packs a powerful punch. That's because fruits and veggies begin to lose their nutrients once they're picked. The sooner you can get your hands on those tomatoes or strawberries, the better.

Don't cast aside cans. If farm fresh is not an option, consider canned. A study published in the *Journal of the Science of Food and Agriculture* shows canned peaches have more vitamin C, antioxidants, and folate than fresh ones. Researchers believe it's because canned peaches are picked and packed as soon as they're ripe. And canning makes nutrients in peaches burst out of cell walls.

Mix up your cooking methods. When it comes to cooking vegetables, what works to keep one vitamin intact may not work for another. Experts say whatever method works for you — baking, boiling, steaming, grilling, or microwaving — that's the one you should choose. But keep frying to a minimum. It's the worst way to preserve nutrients.

Use the following tips to safeguard nutrients as long as possible.

- Store fruits and vegetables in a cool room or in your refrigerator once ripe.
- Place spinach, broccoli, and salad greens in your refrigerator's high-humidity drawer.

- Put canned goods in a cool place and use the liquid when cooking.
- Keep cooking and reheating times to a minimum, and use as little water as possible.
- Leave the skins on fruits and veggies when cooking. You'll find loads of nutrients just under the skin.

Vitamins: are you getting enough?

Vitamin A (fat soluble) aka* Retinol, Retinoic acid	
What it does	controls eyesight, builds new cells, protects skin and mucous membranes, fights infection and free radicals
Signs of deficiency	weak immune system, night blindness, diarrhea, and dry skin and hair
RDA (M)* 14 – 70 yrs.	900 mcg or 3,000 IU
RDA (F)* 14 – 70 yrs.	700 mcg or 2,333 IU
Diet suggestions	1 baked sweet potato (21,909 IU) 1 cup kale, cooked (17,707 IU) 1/2 cup carrots, cooked (13,286 IU)

Vitamin D (fat soluble) aka Calciferol	
What it does	builds bones, controls calcium and phosphorus levels in your body
Signs of deficiency	joint pain, bowing legs, and muscle spasms
RDA (M)* 14 – 70 yrs.	15 mcg or 600 IU
Diet suggestions	3 oz. canned Sockeye salmon, drained (649 IU) 3 oz. canned tuna, in oil and drained (201 IU) 1 cup All-bran cereal with extra fiber (109 IU)

Vitamin E (fat soluble) aka Alpha tocopherol	
What it does	fights free radicals
Signs of deficiency	weakness, leg cramps, pale skin
RDA (M & F) 14 – >70 yrs.	15 mcg
Diet suggestions	1 cup Multi-grain Cheerios (14 mg) 2 Tbsps. smooth peanut butter, vitamin and mineral fortified (14 mg) 2 oz. plain wheat germ, toasted (9 mg)

Vitamin K (fat soluble) aka Phylloquinone	
What it does	forms blood clots, controls calcium levels
Signs of deficiency	excessive bleeding, unknown bruises
AI (M) 19 – >70 yrs.	120 mcg
AI (F) 19 – >70 yrs.	90 mcg
Diet suggestions	1 cup cooked collards, from frozen (1,060 mcg) 1 cup cooked spinach, from frozen (1,028 mcg) 1 cup cooked Brussels sprouts, from frozen (300 mcg)

Warning: If you take blood-thinning drugs (such as warfarin), you may need to limit vitamin K foods.

Vitamin B1 (water soluble) aka Thiamin	
What it does	produces energy, sends nerve messages, brings on healthy appetite
Signs of deficiency	swollen and puffy skin (edema), tiredness, depression, and trouble concentrating
RDA (M) 14 – >70 yrs.	1.2 mg
RDA (F) 19 – >70 yrs.	1.1 mg
Diet suggestions	3/4 cup Wheaties cereal (.7 mg) 1 cup black beans, cooked (.4 mg) 1 cup edamame, cooked (.3 mg)

Vitamin B2 (water soluble) aka Riboflavin	
What it does	produces energy, helps vision, builds new cells
Signs of deficiency	cracked lips, skin rash, trouble seeing in bright light
RDA (M) 14 – >70 yrs.	1.3 mg
RDA (F) 19 – >70 yrs.	1.1 mg
Diet suggestions	1 cup Total Raisin Bran cereal (1.7 mg) 1 cup diced Portabello mushrooms (.4 mg) 1 oz. (approx. 23) almonds (.3 mg)

Vitamin B3 (water soluble) aka Niacin	
What it does	produces energy, builds DNA
Signs of deficiency	diarrhea, black and smooth tongue, trouble concentrating, skin rash
RDA (M) 14 – >70 yrs.	16 mg
RDA (F) 14 – >70 yrs.	14 mg
Diet suggestions	1 cup Special K cereal (7.1 mg) 1 cup lentils, cooked (2.1 mg) 2 slices chicken breast, cooked (1.4 mg)

Folate (water soluble) aka Folic acid, Folacin	
What it does	makes and repairs DNA, removes homocysteine from blood
Signs of deficiency	tiredness, depression, smooth and sore tongue, digestion problems, headaches
RDA (M & F) 14 – >70 yrs.	400 mcg
Diet suggestions	2 oz. garbanzo beans, canned (38 mcg) 1 cup lima beans, cooked (156 mcg) 1 Alaskan King Crab leg, cooked (68 mcg)

Vitamin B12 (water soluble) aka Cobalamin	
What it does	makes new cells (especially red blood cells), protects nerves
Signs of deficiency	numbness in extremities, muscle weakness, weight loss, depression, and smooth or sore tongue
RDA (M & F) 14 – >70 yrs.	2.4 mcg
Diet suggestions	3 oz. ground beef, 80% lean, cooked (2.1 mcg) 1 whole egg, hard-boiled (.6 mcg) 1 cup cottage cheese, 1% fat (1.4 mcg)

Vitamin B6 (water soluble) aka Pyridoxine	
What it does	makes red blood cells, builds proteins, regulates blood sugar, makes brain chemicals, and protects immune system
Signs of deficiency	fatigue, poor moods, smooth or sore tongue, and skin inflammation
RDA (M) 14 – 50 yrs.	1.3 mg
RDA (M) 51 – >70 yrs.	1.7 mg
RDA (F) 19 – 50 yrs.	1.3 mg
RDA (F) 51 – >70 yrs.	1.5 mg
Diet suggestions	1 baked potato (.9 mg) 1 banana (.4 mg) 3 oz. beef tenderloin (.5 mg)

Biotin (water soluble)	
What it does	produces energy, helps body use other B vitamins
Signs of deficiency	loss of appetite, depression, weakness, rash, and hair loss
AI (M & F) 19 – >70 yrs.	30 mcg
Diet suggestions	1/2 cup oats for oatmeal (16 mcg) 1 cup tomatoes, fresh (7 mcg) 1/4 cup walnuts (6 mcg)

Vitamin B5 (water soluble) aka Pantothenic acid	
What it does	produces energy
Signs of deficiency	nausea, insomnia, and tiredness
AI (M & F) 14 – >70 yrs.	5 mg
Diet suggestions	4 oz. sunflower seeds, roasted (8 mg) 4 shiitake mushrooms, dried (3 mg) 2 oz. wheat germ cereal (.8 mg)

Vitamin C (water soluble) aka Ascorbic acid	
What it does	makes collagen for skeleton and skin, fights free radicals, bolsters immune system, helps body absorb iron
Signs of deficiency	bleeding gums, weak bones and joints, blotchy skin, unhealed wounds
RDA (M) 19 – >70 yrs.	90 mg
RDA (F) 19 – >70 yrs.	75 mg
Diet suggestions	1 cup sweet red peppers, chopped (190 mg) 1 cup strawberries, halved (89 mg) 1 cup broccoli florets (66 mg)

*(M) = Males *(F) = Females *aka = also known as
*RDA = Recommended Dietary Allowances *AI = Adequate Intake

Major-league minerals: all-star lineup for super health

Mind your minerals, heal your body

You don't just need vitamins for good health. Minerals are just as important. These elements are found in soil and water. They make their way into your body via the fish, plants, and meats you eat, and the liquids you drink.

Scientists divide minerals into two groups — major and trace. Major minerals include calcium, chloride, phosphorus, potassium, sodium, sulfur, and magnesium. Your body needs all of these to maintain good health.

But don't knock trace minerals — iodine, iron, zinc, selenium, fluoride, chromium, copper, molybdenum, and manganese. Just because your body only needs tiny amounts of trace minerals doesn't mean they're not as important as the major ones.

Minerals work much like the pump and radiator in your car's engine. Sodium, chloride, and potassium regulate your body's water. Calcium, phosphorus, and magnesium promote healthy bones. And sulfur stabilizes the proteins your body needs for healthy hair, skin, and nails.

And don't forget your brain — minerals charge up your brain like a car battery charges a car. Take magnesium, for example. It guards against memory loss. An animal study from China suggests magnesium threonate, a specially formulated compound, may even reverse the cognitive decline associated with Alzheimer's. A more recent human study shows magnesium threonate supplements increase thinking and reasoning skills and decrease forgetfulness.

Potassium from sources like bananas and potatoes maintain your blood pressure, which protects the lining of the arteries in your brain.

A study published in *Nutrition Journal* says iron supplements could boost your IQ and your ability to pay attention and concentrate. But bear in mind, too much iron can be toxic. Adults over age 65 generally have plenty of iron stored in their bodies. So don't take an iron supplement without checking with your doctor first.

Salt shakedown: new health dangers revealed

You can fork over big bucks for a container of exotic salt, but why bother? All salt is created equal, no matter how fancy the label is.

Take sea salt, for instance. Some people think it's better for them, because it's less processed. But sea salt and table salt have the same amount of sodium, so don't think you're eating healthier because you've switched over. The truth is, most salt comes from the sea anyway. To gain any health benefit, you need to focus on the amount of salt you're getting, not the source.

Too much salt can worsen kidney disease, diabetes, congestive heart failure, and osteoporosis. And there's more. Here's a look at two other ways salt sabotages your health.

Autoimmune disorders. Three new studies suggest salt may prompt several autoimmune diseases including psoriasis, multiple sclerosis, rheumatoid arthritis, and ankylosing spondylitis or arthritis of the spine. Yale School of Medicine researchers discovered the link between a high-salt diet and autoimmune conditions when they conducted an animal study. They say too much salt caused the animals to produce inflammatory cells closely associated with autoimmune diseases. These cells attack healthy tissue.

Heart. Researchers say eating too much salt may lead to well over 1 million deaths worldwide every year. That's because salt makes your body retain water, and that raises the amount of blood in your arteries. It also makes small arteries constrict, so your blood strains to get through. High blood pressure is the result, which increases your risk of heart disease and stroke.

Scientists came to these conclusions after gathering information from over 60 countries. But the Institute of Medicine says more research needs to be done to see if less salt in your diet lowers your risk of heart disease.

You don't want to cut salt out of your diet completely. Your body needs sodium to contract muscles, send and receive nerve signals, and regulate fluids and electrolytes. But the American diet is loaded with salt. A committee of nutrition experts from the Food and Nutrition Board set the following Adequate Intakes (AI) for sodium — 1,500 mg/day for ages 19–50, 1,300 mg/day for ages 51–70, and 1,200 mg/day for people over age 70.

Not everyone is as sensitive to salt as others. But experts say if you have diabetes, high blood pressure, chronic kidney disease, are over age 51, or African-American you should definitely cut back. One way to do that is to roast or caramelize foods when you cook. This gives your taste buds the impression that you're eating something salty. So does eating tomatoes, onions, and mushrooms. Or try adding herbs and spices to your dishes like Mrs. Dash, garlic, turmeric, rosemary, and cinnamon. Your taste buds will be happy — and so will your heart.

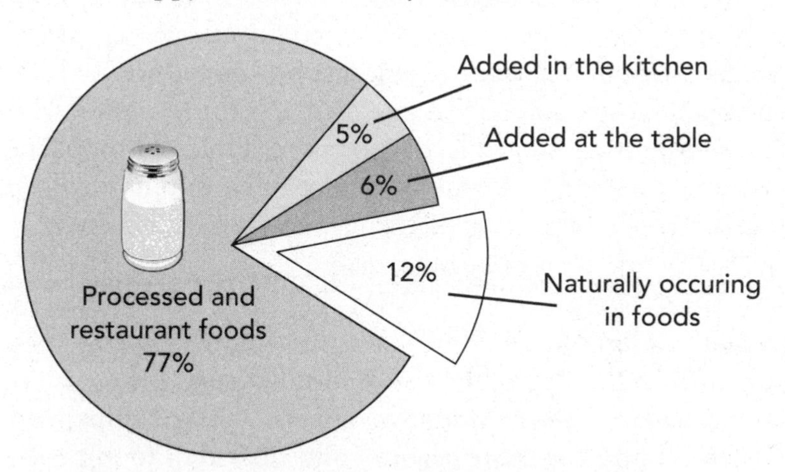

You control over 88% of the salt in your diet.

3 things you need to know about calcium

You think of healthy bones when you think of calcium. And while this mighty mineral certainly does promote strong bones, in some cases it can do more harm than good.

Encourages kidney stones. You wouldn't think calcium and kidney stones would have a link. But they do. A study published in the journal *Menopause* found excess calcium in the blood and urine of women ages 57 to 90. These women added 200 milligrams of a calcium citrate supplement to their diet, taking in a total of 1,200 milligrams a day. They also took between 400 and 4,800 international units (IU) of vitamin D a day. Vitamin D helps your body absorb calcium.

A small number of participants showed excess calcium in their blood, and about one-third had a surplus of calcium in their urine. Doctors fear this excess calcium could play a role in the development of kidney stones in women. But they're not sure why.

Since doctors often recommend 1,200 milligrams of calcium and 400 to 800 (IU) of vitamin D to postmenopausal women, more research needs to be done to understand the link.

Offers little protection against brittle bones. Postmenopausal women run the risk of osteoporosis — weak, fragile bones, and the loss of bone mass. Some people think taking calcium supplements prevents osteoporosis. But research says otherwise. Lots of factors contribute to osteoporosis like race, genes, gender, smoking, body size, exercise, and estrogen levels. So taking a calcium supplement alone won't help. Some experts believe calcium plus estrogen, exercise, and vitamin D supplements may be more effective.

Fortunately, the latest news about calcium isn't all bad.

Clobbers colon cancer. Check out this winning formula — calcium from food plus fiber from food equals a lower risk of colon cancer. A 12-year study with over 1,500 participants out of Poland found the more calcium and fiber-rich food people ate, the lower their chances of developing colon cancer.

Ultimately, doctors suggest you get all of your calcium from foods. And if you think you're not getting enough, assess your diet and calcium intake first. Then talk with your doctor about taking a supplement.

Minerals: are you getting enough?

Calcium (major mineral)	
What it does	builds bones and teeth, contracts muscles and nerves, sends nerve messages, and controls blood pressure
Signs of deficiency	bone loss (osteoporosis)
RDA (M)* 19 – 70 yrs.	1,000 mg
RDA (M) >70 yrs.	1,200 mg
RDA (F)* 19 – 50 yrs.	1,000 mg
RDA (F) 51 – >70 yrs.	1,200 mg
Diet suggestions	2 slices Swiss cheese (442 mg) 4 sardines (183 mg) 1 cup navy beans, cooked (126 mg)

Chloride (major mineral)	
What it does	makes stomach juices for digestion and balances levels of other minerals
Signs of deficiency	muscle cramps, trouble concentrating and loss of appetite
AI (M) 14 – 50 yrs.	2.3 g
AI (M) 51 – 70 yrs.	2.0 g
AI (M) >70 yrs.	1.8 g
AI (F) 14 – 50 yrs.	2.3 g
AI (F) 51 – 70 yrs.	2.0 g
AI (F) >70 yrs.	1.8 g
Diet suggestions	obtained mostly from sodium chloride (table salt)

Magnesium (major mineral)	
What it does	builds bones and teeth, relaxes muscles, makes proteins, helps body use nutrients, and steadies heart rhythm
Signs of deficiency	tiredness, loss of appetite, muscle cramps and twitches, convulsions, depression, and confusion
RDA (M) 31 – >70 yrs.	420 mg
RDA (F) 31 – >70 yrs.	320 mg
Diet suggestions	1 cup quinoa, cooked (118 mg) 1 oz. Brazil nuts (106 mg) 1/4 cup toasted wheat bran (97 mg)

Phosphorus (major mineral)	
What it does	builds new cells and produces energy
Signs of deficiency	loss of appetite, tiredness, and pain in bones
RDA (M & F) 19 – >70 yrs.	700 mg
Diet suggestions	2 slices American cheese (312 mg) 2 Tbsp. almond butter (167 mg) 1 oz. cashew nuts (166 mg)

Potassium (major mineral)	
What it does	sends nerve messages, relaxes nerves, maintains chemical balances, and steadies blood pressure
Signs of deficiency	dehydration, weakness, and trouble concentrating
AI (M & F) 14 – >70 yrs.	4.7 g
Diet suggestions	1 cup Great Northern beans, cooked (692 mg) 1 baked sweet potato (541 mg) 1/4 cup dried apricots (378 mg)

Sodium (major mineral)	
What it does	balances fluid levels and sends nerve messages
Signs of deficiency	muscle cramps, trouble concentrating, and loss of appetite
AI (M & F) 9 – 50 yrs.	1.5 g or 1,500 mg
AI (M & F) 51 – 70 yrs.	1.3 g or 1,300 mg
Diet sources high in sodium	1 tsp. table salt (2,325 mg) 10 pretzel twists, salted (1,029 mg) 1 cup Campbell's chicken noodle soup (1,780 mg)

Sulfur (major mineral)	
What it does	builds vitamins and proteins and removes toxic chemicals
Signs of deficiency	protein deficiency
RDA (M & F)	unknown
Diet sources high in sulfur amino acids and compounds	protein-rich food like cow's milk, eggs, meats, and also cruciferous vegetables

Boron (trace mineral)	
What it does	helps body use calcium and builds bones and joints
Signs of deficiency	bone loss (osteoporosis) and joint pain (osteoarthritis)
RDA (M & F)	unknown
Diet suggestions	1 small box of raisins (2 mg) 1/2 cup prunes, stewed (1.5 mg) 35 hazelnuts (1.4 mg)

Chromium (trace mineral)	
What it does	produces energy and balances blood sugar level
Signs of deficiency	high blood sugar level
AI (M) 14 – 50 yrs.	35 mcg
AI (M) 51 – >70 yrs.	30 mcg
AI (F) 19 – 50 yrs.	25 mcg
AI (F) 51 – >70 yrs.	20 mcg
Diet suggestions	1/2 cup broccoli (11 mcg) 1 cup grape juice (8 mcg) 1 whole-wheat English muffin (4 mcg)

Copper (trace mineral)	
What it does	makes red blood cells, produces energy, and fights free radicals
Signs of deficiency	weakness, pale skin, and unhealed wounds
RDA (M & F) 19 – >70 yrs.	900 mcg
Diet suggestions	6 oysters, moist heat (3.2 mg) 3 Tbsp. sesame seeds (1.2 mg) 2 Tbsp. cashew butter (.8 mg)

Fluoride (trace mineral)	
What it does	protects bones and teeth
Signs of deficiency	dental cavities
AI (M) 19 – >70 yrs.	4 mg
AI (F) 14 – >70 yrs.	3 mg
Diet suggestions	1 cup brewed tea, with tap water (884 mcg) 1 6-oz. can of crabmeat, drained (262 mcg) 1 cup brewed coffee, with tap water (215 mcg)

Iodine (trace mineral)	
What it does	makes thyroid hormones and steadies metabolism
Signs of deficiency	goiter
RDA (M & F) 14 – >70 yrs.	150 mcg
Diet suggestions	4 oz. scallops (135 mcg) 1 cup yogurt (71 mcg) 1 cup milk (56 mcg)

Iron (trace mineral)	
What it does	carries oxygen throughout body and produces energy
Signs of deficiency	weakness, pale skin, and trouble concentrating
RDA (M) 19 – >70 yrs.	8 mg
RDA (F) 19 – 50 yrs.	18 mg
RDA (F) 51 – >70 yrs.	8 mg
Diet suggestions	1/2 pkg. or 5.5 oz. dried fruit mix, prune, apricot, and pear (8 mg) 1 cup red kidney beans, cooked (5 mg) 2 hard-boiled eggs (1 mg)

Manganese (trace mineral)	
What it does	produces energy, builds bones, and joints
Signs of deficiency	unknown
AI (M) 19 – >70 yrs.	2.3 mg
AI (F) 19 – >70 yrs.	1.8 mg
Diet suggestions	1 Tbsp. wheat germ (2.7 mg) 3 Tbsp. chickpeas (.9 mg) 22 almonds (.7 mg)

Molybdenum (trace mineral)	
What it does	fights free radicals
Signs of deficiency	severe headache, rapid heartbeat, and confusion
RDA (M & F) 19 – >70 yrs.	45 mcg
Diet suggestions	1 cup navy beans (196 mcg) 1 cup lentils (148 mcg) 1 cup peanuts (42 mcg)

Selenium (trace mineral)	
What it does	makes thyroid hormones, fights free radicals, and strengthens immune system
Signs of deficiency	muscle weakness and pain, cataracts, and heart trouble
RDA (M & F) 14 – >70 yrs.	55 mcg
Diet suggestions	3 oz. sockeye salmon (64 mcg) 1/4 cup mixed nuts (50 mcg) 1 cup amaranth flakes (27 mcg)

Zinc (trace mineral)	
What it does	produces energy, makes DNA, helps body use vitamin A, fights free radicals, heals wounds, and boosts immune system
Signs of deficiency	diarrhea, infections, loss of appetite, weight loss, and unhealed wounds
RDA (M) 14 – >70 yrs.	11 mg
RDA (F) 19 – >70 yrs.	8 mg
Diet suggestions	1 cup Multi-grain Cheerios (16 mg) 2 Tbsp. creamy peanut butter, vitamin and mineral fortified (5 mg) 1 oz. (about 85) pumpkin seeds (3 mg)

*(M) = Males *(F) = Females *aka = also known as
*DRI = Dietary Reference Intake *AI = Adequate Intake

Phytochemicals: nutrients that keep you young

Powerful plant chemicals wage war on disease

You've heard the phrase "them's fightin' words." Think of phytochemicals the same way — fighting chemicals that clobber cancer and pump up your immune system.

Also known as phytonutrients, they give plants their scents, colors, and flavors. Here's a quick look at how phytochemicals will put up their dukes for you.

- Block cancer-causing substances in the food you eat and air you breathe.
- Lower the inflammation that triggers cancer cell growth.
- Curb the growth rate of cancer cells.
- Help your body regulate hormones.
- Lower blood pressure, fight bad bacteria, and reduce cholesterol.

Maybe you've seen the words carotenoids, flavonoids, and resveratrol, but aren't sure what they are. These are examples of some better known phytochemicals. You can find them in peanuts, oregano, fruits, whole grains, teas, wines, and grape juice.

You don't need phytochemicals to stay alive like you do other nutrients. But with all of their amazing health benefits, why not let these super sluggers fight for your health.

Boost your brain with a tiny berry

I'll bet you didn't know you don't have to lose your memories — blueberries can keep your brain sharp.

That's because blueberries are loaded with phytochemicals called anthocyanins. These nutrients give berries their vibrant red, blue, and purple colors. And they boost your brain power thanks to their antioxidant and anti-inflammatory properties.

Researchers found that women who ate blueberries at least once a week suffered less memory loss than those who didn't. The study, published in the *Annals of Neurology*, looked at the eating habits of more than 16,000 women ages 70 and up over 20-plus years. Participants ate a half cup of blueberries or two half-cup servings of strawberries a week. The women who ate the most berries suffered the least memory loss.

You don't just have to eat blueberries to benefit from anthocyanins. Enjoy blueberry juice. It's the "must drink" juice for anyone over age 50 because it improves brain function and mood even in folks with memory problems. Experts at the University of Cincinnati Academic Health Center asked older adults with early memory problems to drink about two cups of wild blueberry juice every day for 12 weeks. The small study showed a marked improvement in the participants' ability to learn and recall word lists. Scientists believe blueberry juice could help adults at risk of dementia.

Researchers aren't sure why anthocyanins help with memory and brain function. But they think these mighty nutrients revive nerve cells and help them send each other signals that help you learn and remember.

Experts also say freezing blueberries not only preserves their antioxidants — it makes them more available. That's because freezing raises the concentration of anthocyanins in berries. So top your pancakes or oatmeal with fresh blueberries, toss frozen ones in a smoothie, or enjoy a refreshing glass of blueberry juice. Your brain will never forget these delicious treats.

Go nuts for greater brainpower

It takes just seven to improve your balance, coordination, and memory. Seven servings? Ounces? No — just seven little nuts. All you have to do is snack on walnuts to keep your brain sharp.

Walnuts are brimming with polyphenols — phytochemicals with antioxidant properties. An animal study from Tufts University found snacking on walnuts improved balance, coordination, and memory in older subjects. Past studies have shown these benefits from fruits and vegetables. But now walnuts, eaten in moderation, can be added to the list.

A human study published in the *Journal of Nutrition* shows eating walnuts boosts memory, processing speed, and reasoning and thinking skills. Experts believe it's because polyphenols spark nerve cell activity and lower inflammation, delivering the charge your brain needs to stay sharp.

Sprinkle walnuts over yogurt, toss in a salad, or blend into low-fat cream cheese for a tasty snack.

3 great reasons to take time for tea

Legend has it Chinese emperor Shen Nung discovered tea in 2737 B.C. when tea leaves blew off a tree and into a pot of boiling water. While the legend may or may not be true, scientists today know one thing for sure — tea boasts tremendous health perks.

Green tea packs a powerful combination of caffeine and phytochemicals called catechins. Studies show green tea drinkers lost fat, raised their metabolism rate, and lowered their cholesterol — just by drinking several cups every day. Researchers believe it's the epigallocatechin gallate (EGCG) — a catechin found in green tea — that makes it stand out from the rest.

Observational studies from several countries and cultures, like Japan, show a link between low cancer rates and high consumption of green tea. Other research suggests green tea may lower the inflammation associated with inflammatory bowel disease and help control blood sugar levels in people with type 1 diabetes. And there are other ways green tea can benefit you.

Whittles your waist. Studies show drinking four cups of green tea a day helps people lose weight and trim inches from their waist. One study published in the *Journal of Research in Medical Sciences* found these results to be true with overweight participants. Experts say EGCG boosts your body's ability to burn calories and fat.

Lowers your blood pressure. Several Japanese studies show lower blood pressure in green tea drinkers, especially older women who drank four cups a day. The phytochemicals in green tea seem to keep your heart and the inner lining of your blood vessels healthy.

Boots bad cholesterol. Drinking tea may also lower your LDL cholesterol. A review of 14 trials with more than 1,100 people found green tea can lower your bad cholesterol by 5 to 6 points. The findings were published in the *American Journal of Clinical Nutrition.* Researchers think it's because catechins cause your gut to absorb less cholesterol.

Super charge your heart with flavonoids

Looking for a way to strengthen and protect your heart? Look no further than foods brimming with flavonoids.

You get flavonoids from plant-based foods, just like all other phytochemicals. But flavonoids, in particular, seem to boost your health and battle diseases more so than other phytochemicals. Plus, they safeguard your heart in a number of ways.

Battle high blood pressure. No one wants to deal with high blood pressure, especially since it increases your risk for serious health problems, like heart disease and stroke.

Eating a cup of blueberries a week may help. In fact, fresh, frozen, canned, or jellied, this common fruit helps protect your eyes, heart, and veins.

A study published in the *American Journal of Clinical Nutrition* of more than 87,000 people shows participants who ate the most blueberries and strawberries had the lowest risk of developing high blood pressure. Experts say you can thank the anthocyanins and other flavonoids in berries. These nutrients open up blood vessels, making it easier for blood to flow and keeping blood pressure in a healthy range.

Plus, the active ingredients in blueberries may boost your eyesight. In an animal study from China Agricultural University, researchers found a diet that included wild Chinese blueberries healed retinal damage caused by exposure to too much light.

Repair damage to blood vessels. Dark chocolate could save your life. That's because this melt-in-your-mouth treat is loaded with flavanols — flavonoids that topple high blood pressure and pump up your good cholesterol.

What's more, research from the University of California shows cocoa flavanols could repair damaged blood vessels. Researchers think it's because cocoa flavanols boost the number of circulating angiogenic cells (CACs) in the blood. CACs keep blood vessels healthy and repair those that are damaged. And the more CACs you have, the lower your chances of dying from heart-related problems, suggests a study published in the *New England Journal of Medicine*.

Flush out arteries. You need healthy arteries for a healthy heart. You can keep your arteries young with one delicious fruit juice — cranberry. This tart and tasty berry juice overflows with

A-type proanthocyanidins — phytochemicals not found in most other berries.

- Several animal and human studies suggest the active ingredients in cranberry juice lower bad LDL cholesterol and raise good HDL cholesterol.
- Additional human studies show cranberry anthocyanins lower the inflammation that can lead to atherosclerosis — or hardening of the arteries.
- Cranberry's phytochemicals help keep your arteries flexible so they can transport blood with ease.

Cranberry juice isn't the only beverage loaded with perks. You can have cleaner arteries in four weeks just by drinking tea. A study from Boston University School of Medicine suggests drinking black tea could promote heart health. Researchers think tea's flavonoids make arteries work better.

Foil heart disease. Olive oil can actually lubricate your blood vessels, keeping blood flowing freely. This delicious oil will keep your arteries from hardening. One study published in the *European Journal of Nutrition* found the catechins in olive oil improved artery function in people with early signs of atherosclerosis.

Another study suggests olive oil may trigger antibodies that stop oxidized LDL cholesterol from damaging artery walls, thereby lowering your risk for atherosclerosis.

Guard against heart attacks. You know them, you love them — apples. This one fruit is a heart-attack stopper — as much as a 23 percent drop in bad cholesterol in just one year.

A Florida State University study of women ages 45 to 65 surprised researchers. Scientists did not expect bad cholesterol numbers to nosedive after just six months in women who ate dried apples daily. Plus, the tart treat raised their good cholesterol.

And the women lost weight, even though the apples added an extra 240 calories to their daily intake. Researchers think the flavonoids in apples boost fat burning.

Unconventional ways to keep your bones strong

Sticks and stones may break your bones, but this sweet snack and comforting drink will never hurt you.

Dried plums. A prune a day may keep constipation at bay. And it's also the fruit that doesn't just slow bone loss — it reverses it.

A recent animal study shows that prunes, also known as dried plums, prevent bone loss and restore bones. Scientists think it's the polyphenols and their antioxidant and anti-inflammatory properties that promote bone health.

A recent animal study shows postmenopausal women who ate dried plums regularly had a lower chance of developing osteoporosis or fractures than those who didn't eat them. Some researchers believe dried plums are the world's easiest way to keep your bones strong.

"I have tested numerous fruits, including figs, dates, strawberries and raisins," said Professor Bahram H. Arjmandi of Florida State University, "and none of them come anywhere close to having the effect on bone density that dried plums, or prunes, have."

Green tea. Battle brittle bone disease with a tasty cup of this — and it's not milk. It's green tea, a refreshing drink brimming with polyphenols.

Researchers in Hong Kong found that an active ingredient in green tea called epigallocatechin (EGC) made bones stronger. Lab studies also show EGC boosts a key enzyme that promotes bone growth by up to 79 percent. And a review of scientific research conducted by a team of experts suggests green tea may prevent age-related bone loss and the risk of fractures in elderly men and women. Scientists say they believe it's the polyphenols in green tea that seem to benefit bones, but more research needs to be done.

Make no bones about it — a delicious cup of green tea and a handful of dried plums will give your bones the boost they need to stay strong.

Savory spice helps prevent 8 types of cancer

Multitalented turmeric, an ingredient in curry, gives Indian dishes their bright yellow coloring, serves up a healthy dose of the phytochemical curcumin, and helps kiss cancer good-bye.

Colon. Curcumin keeps blood vessels from providing oxygen and nutrients to cancer cells and might also charge up vitamin D in the colon where experts say it acts as a cancer-fighting agent.

Breast. Research published in the journal *Breast Cancer Research and Treatment* says curcumin may prevent breast cancer cells from forming, growing, and spreading. And a review of several studies published in *Integrative Biology* says curcumin shows promise as a way to prevent breast cancer. But if you already have breast cancer, talk with your doctor. Some studies suggest curcumin interferes with cyclophosphamide, a chemotherapy drug.

Prostate. This cancer takes several years to kick into full gear and is often related to a high-fat diet, lack of exercise — and inflammation. But curcumin seems to halt the inflammation that can lead to prostate cancer.

Brain. Experts from MD Anderson Cancer Center say curcumin prevents brain cancer cells from growing and spreading, and encourages the death of cancer cells.

Leukemia. When someone has leukemia, or cancer of the blood cells, their bone marrow produces abnormal white blood cells. Called leukemia cells, they grow fast and crowd out normal blood cells. Scientists think curcumin triggers an excessive production of reactive oxygen species — molecules that promote leukemia cell death.

Melanoma. This skin cancer is the deadliest of all skin cancers. But a recent German study suggests curcumin inhibits the growth of melanoma cancer cells.

Pancreatic. Cook up curcumin with olive oil for a tasty way to block pancreatic cancer. A study published in the journal *Nutrition and Cancer* suggests the combination of curcumin and omega-3 fatty acids may prevent, battle, and kill pancreatic cancer cells.

Head and neck. Scientists believe the golden spice shuts down the communication between cells that trigger cancer cell growth. It also lowers the number of pro-inflammatory cytokines — substances that promote inflammation and cancer growth. Many experts suggest taking curcumin as a supplement, because you can't get the amount you need to fight head and neck cancer from spicing up your food.

If beating eight kinds of cancer isn't enough, the dynamic spice eases joint pain, too. Several promising studies suggest curcumin works as an anti-inflammatory by blocking a protein that triggers inflammation.

2 simple ways to outsmart breast cancer

A big bowl of blackberries could better your odds of beating breast cancer and slash your chances of getting it in the first place. That's because blackberries are loaded with cancer-fighting nutrients called phytoestrogens.

Researchers first observed phytoestrogens in plants in the 1920s and noticed they act a lot like estrogens — hence the name. And in recent studies, scientists have focused on the phytoestrogens in lignans and cruciferous veggies, and have discovered the reason why these two types of foods curb the development and spread of cancers.

Lignans. There's a relationship between estrogen and breast cancer — and it's not a romantic one. Researchers at Cornell University found that women who got breast cancer had more estrogen circulating through their bodies than women without it. Another study shows that women treated for breast cancer who had high levels of estrogen got it again sooner than breast cancer survivors with low estrogen levels.

But a study published in the *American Journal of Clinical Nutrition* suggests lignans lower the odds of breast cancer in postmenopausal women. Scientists say it's because the phytoestrogen in lignans — enterolactone — binds with estrogens, keeping them from wreaking havoc on breast cells.

Besides blackberries, add lignans to your diet by eating kale, ground flaxseeds, garlic, raspberries, and pomegranates.

Cruciferous vegetables. You know broccoli is good for you, but just how good? Good enough to beat breast cancer. A Swedish study of over 5,000 postmenopausal women shows that those who ate one or two servings of cruciferous vegetables daily lowered their risk of breast cancer by as much as 40 percent. Experts believe the phytochemical indole-3-carbinol in broccoli, cabbage, cauliflower, and other cruciferous vegetables prevents cancer by squashing free radicals, changing estrogen into a form that's less-likely to cause cancer, and partly blocking estrogen's effect on cells.

Some experts have examined other studies and disagree. They argue the research is not consistent and say more studies need to be done.

Regardless, eating lignans and cruciferous vegetables is one delicious way to stay healthy. So why not ramp up your servings of blackberries and broccoli? They will do your body good.

Save your eyesight, no matter your age

A whopping 20 million Americans over age 18 can't see clearly. And the older you get, the worse your vision gets. But two phytochemicals — lutein and zeaxanthin — can save your eyes from two sight stealers.

These powerful nutrients slash the risk of vision loss from age-related macular degeneration (AMD) and cataracts. Experts say it's because lutein and zeaxanthin protect your eyes from sunlight and other damage.

AMD. This condition affects the macula, the central part of the retina that helps you see what's directly in front of you. Scientists don't know why the macula's health fades as you get older. But the Age-Related Eye Disease Study (AREDS and AREDS2) sheds light on what you can do about it.

Adding lutein and zeaxanthin lowered the risk of advanced AMD in two groups — participants whose diets were already low in the two phytochemicals and those who took an antioxidant supplement without beta-carotene.

Go green to boost your lutein and zeaxanthin — kale, green peas, spinach, collards, and turnip greens are packed with these powerful phytochemicals.

Cataracts. Scientists aren't sure why the proteins in your eyes clump together to form a cataract and blurry vision. But they do know certain nutrients can help lower your risk.

In the AREDS2 study, participants who didn't regularly eat a lot of foods with lutein and zeaxanthin lowered their risk of developing cataracts by adding the phytochemicals in supplement form to their diet.

A review of several studies published in the *British Journal of Nutrition* also shows that eating foods rich in lutein and zeaxanthin lowered the risk of cataracts in older women.

And the Health Professional's Follow-up Study from Harvard found eating about 7 milligrams of foods rich in lutein and zeaxanthin every day reduced the need for cataract surgery. That's just under two cups of raw spinach or green peas.

Big benefits from 5 little-known nutrients

Many phytochemicals make headlines. Others you never hear about, but they're just as important for your health. Here's a look at a few of them and their powerful perks.

Limonene. This tangy nutrient clobbers cancer cells and keeps them from spreading. You find these in lime, lemon, orange, grapefruit, and tangerine peels. But if eating peels doesn't sound, well, appealing, you can toss lemon zest into pasta, make candied peels, or create your own citrus salt.

Sterols and stanols. They look like cholesterol but do more good than harm. Plant sterols block bad fats from getting absorbed by your intestines. The results? Lower LDL cholesterol. Add them to your diet by switching over to sterol-fortified spreads or orange juice. Or eat asparagus, nuts and seeds, and whole grains.

Tannins. What do tea, cider, and chickpeas have in common? They all tackle cancer cells and stop them from wreaking havoc with your health. That's because they contain tannins — cancer-fighters with antioxidant abilities.

Organosulfur. If you love the pungent flavors of chives, onions, and garlic, you're in luck. These flavorful foods trigger your body's defenses against cancer. And here's a tip for garlic-lovers. Chopping or crushing garlic 10 minutes before cooking it boosts its cancer-fighting compounds.

Chlorogenic acid. Java lovers take note. Coffee is loaded with chlorogenic acid — a phytochemical that protects your central nervous system from degenerative nerve diseases like Alzheimer's and Parkinson's. And you don't have to drink caffeinated joe for this health perk. Decaf serves up the same protection.

Water: tap into its healing power

Wash away 3 top health hazards

The soda market is tasting a little flat. Water, that wonderfully healthy, natural refreshment, is now the most popular beverage in the United States. Find out why an extra glass of this cheap, beverage may be just what you need to feel better and stay well.

Defends your heart. Your heart pumps blood through your body more easily when you drink enough water. One study even suggests five glasses a day may lower your risk of a heart attack.

So how much should you drink? The Institute of Medicine once recommended 2.7 liters, a little more than 11 cups, of fluids for women, and 3.7 liters, almost 16 cups, for men, but the right amount also depends on things like how much you sweat and how much water you get from moisture-rich foods.

That's why experts no longer recommend eight glasses of water daily. Instead, most healthy people can stay hydrated by drinking water whenever they're thirsty.

Just remember, as you age, your thirst mechanism doesn't work as well as it once did, so don't wait until you're thirsty to drink.

If you're an older adult or have a chronic health condition, like heart disease or diabetes, ask your doctor if drinking more water could help you avoid straining your heart and other organs.

Protects your mood and mind. Even mild dehydration can mean trouble. In a recent study, mildly dehydrated young women had less ability to concentrate, found tasks more difficult, felt more fatigued and angry, and were more prone to headaches. When young men were mildly dehydrated, they became less vigilant, had poorer working memory, and felt more tired and anxious.

Anyone can get mildly dehydrated during a normal day's activities, but older adults and people with diabetes may be even more susceptible. Drink mostly water, but experts now say juice, green tea, and other caffeinated drinks can help you rehydrate, too.

Juices your joints. Water can take the edge off your arthritis and ease a world of hurts. Without enough water, increased friction between joints can mean more swelling, stiffness, and pain. Drink water to lubricate and cushion your joints and transport the nutrients they need.

The buildup of uric acid causes gout, another kind of arthritis. Studies show drinking water flushes out uric acid and helps prevent painful gout attacks.

Enjoying more water may also ease or prevent these health concerns.

- Constipation. Women who consume less liquid are more likely to become constipated, a recent study found.
- High blood sugar and diabetes. Drinking at least 17 ounces of water a day — just over 2 cups — may cut your risk.

Drinking water helps prevent cavities by washing away acid-producing food, and it fights bladder cancer by flushing out cancer-causing substances.

Douse the danger of kidney stones

Director Alfred Hitchcock was in the middle of filming a movie when it happened, and Amazon CEO Jeff Bezos was vacationing on a tropical island. Nobody expects a painful kidney stone, but the odds of getting one have nearly doubled in recent years. Fortunately, this is one problem you can start preventing today.

Get the lowdown on stones. Stones form in your kidneys when you have too much calcium, phosphorus, or oxalate in your urine. The most common stones are a mix of calcium and phosphorus or calcium and oxalate. Tiny stones may pass from your kidneys to your bladder and out of your body without symptoms. But other stones can cause strong pain in your back or lower belly, and possibly nausea and vomiting.

Call your doctor if you have any of these symptoms:

- extreme pain in your back or lower belly that doesn't get better
- blood in your urine
- fever and chills
- vomiting
- urine that smells bad or looks cloudy
- pain when you urinate

Some large stones may get stuck and prevent urine from passing. Doctors remove these stones or break them up so they move out of your body.

Stop stones before they start. Drinking 2 to 3 liters (about 8 to 12 cups) of fluids every day is the best way to prevent kidney stones, but also try these suggestions:

- Avoid sugar-sweetened punch and sodas, especially cola, which raise your odds of stones by up to 33 percent. Experts suspect fructose in these drinks increases the calcium and oxalate in urine. But drinking water, orange juice, and caffeinated or decaf coffee or tea lowers your risk.
- Mix lemon or lime juice with water to make lemonade or limeade, and drink orange juice. The citrate in these juices helps prevent stones.

- Cut back on salt, but be sure you get enough calcium.
- Eat less meat, fish, eggs, and other animal protein.
- Cut back on high-oxalate foods, like nuts, wheat bran, rhubarb, and spinach, or enjoy these foods with milk or other calcium-rich foods or drinks. Oxalate in your kidneys encourages stones to form, but calcium binds oxalate before it reaches your kidneys, reducing the danger of calcium-oxalate stones.
- Exercise regularly. Walking half an hour every day may reduce your risk of stones up to 31 percent.
- Watch your weight and calories. Obesity is linked to higher odds of stones.
- Eat more high-fiber fruits and vegetables. If you're a woman past menopause, that may protect you against kidney stones.

If you've already had a kidney stone, you have a 50 percent chance of having another one, but drinking at least 12 cups of water every day may prevent stones from forming.

Additives: hidden dangers in your food

7 scariest food additives you're eating now

Food companies used an FDA loophole to introduce new food additives that may not be safe, claim public health groups. Food companies deny this, and say ensuring safe products is in their own best interest. So what counts as a food additive, and what does all this mean for you?

Know your additives. During the making or processing of a food, extra ingredients may be added. Any that become part of the final product or affect its characteristics are called food additives. Additives can be natural, like vinegar, salt, or spices, or manmade chemicals, like artificial colors and preservatives.

Additives are used for many good reasons.

- add nutrients
- keep the product fresh
- prevent foodborne illness
- help process or prepare the product
- preserve texture
- enhance color or flavor

Compounds from packaging or other sources may end up in the food unintentionally, but these are also regulated as additives.

Grade the new safety rules. Originally, the FDA required companies to submit rigorous safety research to get a new additive approved. But for approval of common food ingredients, companies only needed to provide research that showed an ingredient was already Generally Recognized as Safe (GRAS). The FDA painstakingly reviewed the research for both GRAS and non-GRAS additives.

But in 1997, the FDA stopped requiring companies to submit research for GRAS products, settling for a research summary instead — and even that was optional. Many companies started submitting nearly all products as GRAS, including non-GRAS additives.

Some companies even declared their products as GRAS without seeking FDA approval. The Pew Charitable Trust estimates approximately 1,000 additives, labeled as GRAS, have been brought to market without being submitted for FDA approval.

In response to a recent lawsuit, the FDA promised to update their rule on the approval process in 2016.

Beware these additives. Experts say salt, sweeteners, and trans fats are the food additives you should worry about most, but you may also want to avoid these.

- Potassium bromate: Banned in other countries, this strengthens and stabilizes bread dough. It has been reduced or eliminated by most bakers.
- BHA (butylated hydroxyanisole) and BHT (butylated hydroxytoluene): Found in cereal, potato chips, gum, and oil, these chemicals prevent oils from becoming rancid, but they may also cause cancer.
- Nitrites and nitrates: These preservatives in packaged meats may help create cancer-causing compounds in your body.
- Sulfites: Found in vinegar, wine, packaged vegetables, and dried fruit, these preservatives may cause headaches or life-threatening reactions in some people with asthma.
- Monosodium glutamate (MSG): This flavor booster is added to many Chinese foods, frozen entrees, salad dressings, chips,

dips, and soups. In large amounts, MSG may cause headaches, muscle aches, and flushing in some people.

- Caramel coloring: Some caramel coloring additives contain 4-methylimidazole (4-MeI), a suspected cancer-causer. Research by *Consumer Reports* suggests some caramel-colored soft drinks may not be safe, but you can't tell which ones. Some suggest avoiding all soft drinks.
- Artificial colors: These may cause allergic reactions in certain people, especially Yellow No. 5 or 6, Red No. 3 or 40, Blue No. 1 or 2, and Green No. 3.

These may not be the only additives to watch out for. Avoiding packaged, processed, and fast foods can help limit or eliminate other potentially unsafe additives.

If you need to avoid a specific food additive due to allergies or other health reasons, check ingredient labels carefully, but be aware that some items may not appear on food labels.

Visit *www.cspinet.org* for more information about individual additives.

Dangers and side effects of artificial sweeteners

Artificial sweeteners won't cause cavities, raise your blood sugar, or add many calories to your diet. They're also super sweet, so you can use less. But some health watchdog groups are concerned about their safety, and the FDA has set Acceptable Daily Intake limits on how much you can consume daily without harm. Cut through the confusion, and make smarter choices with this quick guide to the most common artificial sweeteners.

Acesulfame potassium or acesulfame-K (Sunett, Sweet One). Although the FDA has declared this safe, watchdog groups are calling for new studies about possible thyroid damage and cancer risk, and the Center for Science in the Public Interest (CSPI) recommends you avoid it.

Aspartame (Equal, NutraSweet, Sugar Twin). Foods containing aspartame also include the amino acid phenylalanine, so their labels must include a statement about their phenylalanine content. This helps people who have phenylketonuria — difficulty digesting phenylalanine — avoid it.

Although the FDA declared aspartame safe, the CSPI recommends avoiding it because of concerns about cancer. Some people also report headaches and dizziness that may be related to aspartame.

Advantame. As the newest artificial sweetener approved by the FDA, advantame needs time to develop established brand names. Because advantame is a mix of vanillan and aspartame, it's much sweeter than aspartame. So you need much less to reach your preferred level of sweetness. Because the phenylalanine amounts are so tiny, this sweetener doesn't require special labeling about phenylalanine. Both the FDA and CSPI consider advantame safe.

Saccharin (Sweet'N Low, Sweet Twin). No longer considered a cancer risk, the FDA has approved this sweetener as safe. Yet, the CSPI recommends avoiding it, and some say a 150-pound person should have no more than eight packets a day.

Sucralose (Splenda). Recent, unpublished research suggests sucralose may cause leukemia in mice exposed to the sweetener before birth. CSPI recommends caution with this sweetener, but the FDA says it's safe.

When choosing and using artificial sweeteners, also remember these important points.

- Equal Next, Equal Original, Equal Spoonful, and some soft drinks contain two artificial sweeteners instead of one. Read ingredient labels on all food and drink products to make sure you don't get an artificial sweetener you don't want.

- Most artificial sweeteners are available as tabletop sweeteners and can be used in baking, but aspartame can lose its sweetness at high temperatures. Only add it near the end of cooking.

Keep good foods from going bad

Surprising threats from 5 common foods

One out of every six Americans will get sick from contaminated food or beverages this year, health officials predict. That's nearly 41 million people with the telltale symptoms of diarrhea, nausea, vomiting, and stomach cramps. Roughly 128,000 end up in hospitals, and some never recover. But a few minutes of taking precautions against foodborne illness can save you from days of being sick — or worse.

Start with all the usual safety precautions — like frequent handwashing, proper refrigerator and cooking temperatures, and avoiding cross contamination between foods. But in addition to those, pay special attention to these five foods.

Eggs. Don't wash eggs. The wash water can leak through the eggshell's pores, raising the risk of contamination. And always use a food thermometer to make sure casseroles and other dishes containing eggs are cooked to a temperature of at least 160 degrees. Keep eggs in their carton, not in the refrigerator door's egg slots. Tuck the carton at the back of a shelf to keep eggs at a cold enough temperature to be safe.

Poultry. Don't rinse poultry. The splashes from poultry juices spread bacteria onto nearby kitchen surfaces. Instead, kill those bacteria by cooking the fowl to an internal temperature of 165 degrees. Check the temperature with a meat thermometer to be certain.

Also, take steps to prevent contamination from dripping juices. At the supermarket, put poultry in its own plastic bag, separate from other foods. In the refrigerator, perch the fowl on a tray to keep drippings away from other edibles.

Pork. Buy pork chops instead of ground pork because ground pork is more likely to be contaminated than pork chops. After recent testing, *Consumer Reports* recommends cooking ground pork to an internal temperature of 160 degrees and whole pork to at least 145 degrees. Allow the meat to rest for three minutes after you finish cooking it, or some of the bacteria might survive.

Seafood. Spoiled seafood has an ammonia odor both before and after cooking. Don't buy or eat seafood that smells like ammonia.

Leafy greens. If a package of leafy greens is labeled as prewashed, washing them again won't remove any contaminants. Yet washing uncontaminated, prewashed greens can transfer dangerous bacteria from your hands or kitchen tools to the greens. That's why the FDA advises you to avoid washing bagged greens if they're labeled prewashed and ready-to-eat. Some experts suggest you skip ready-to-eat, bagged and cut greens like lettuce because you can't wash off contaminants if they've worked their way inside cut leaves.

The 5-second rule: fact or fiction

This well-known rule suggests that food you drop on the floor is still safe to eat if you pick it up within five seconds — as long as you rinse it off. Researchers put that to the test in studies, and here's what they found. "A dropped item is immediately contaminated and can't really be sanitized," said Dr. Jorge Parada, medical director of the Infection Prevention and Control Program at Loyola University Health System. "When it comes to folklore, the 'five-second rule' should be replaced with 'When in doubt, throw it out.'"

Going meatless: is it right for you?

4 meaty questions about going vegetarian

Actress and comedian Betty White may be in her 90s, but she's still a walking advertisement for eating a vegetarian diet. Is this diet right for you? Answers to common questions about vegetarianism may help you find out.

What is a vegetarian diet? Vegetarian diets eliminate or restrict meats, including poultry and seafood, and may eliminate other animal products. Instead, vegetarian meals focus on fruits, vegetables, whole grains, seeds, nuts, and legumes. There are several types of vegetarian diets.

- vegan: eliminates any food that comes from animals, including meats, fish, eggs, dairy products, and honey.
- lacto-vegetarian: excludes meats, fish, and eggs, but allows dairy products.
- ovo-vegetarian: eliminates meats, fish, and dairy products, but permits eggs.
- pescetarian: excludes dairy products, eggs, and meats but includes fish.
- flexitarian or semi-vegetarian: allows meat and fish occasionally.

Can it help with my health problems? Two studies suggest a vegan diet can mean lower cholesterol, more weight loss, and less medication for people with chronic diseases. This diet worked even better than the American Diabetes Association diet for people with diabetes.

Vegetarian diets may also help reduce blood pressure and blood sugar. What's more, vegetarian diets may help prevent cancer, obesity, cataracts, metabolic syndrome, and gallstones.

What pitfalls should I watch out for? You must still limit calories and fat, and avoid added oils, fats, and refined carbohydrates — both starches and sweets.

Also, eat a wide variety of foods to avoid nutritional deficiencies. Vegetarians may need to work harder to get enough iron, calcium, vitamin B12, protein, zinc, vitamin D, and omega-3 fatty acids. Eating fortified foods, like cereals and breads, or taking supplements can help, particularly for vitamins B12 and D. But also include foods like beans and nut butter for protein and iron, leafy greens and almonds for calcium, walnuts and flaxseed for omega-3 fatty acids, and white beans and pumpkin seeds for zinc.

Finally, eat combinations of proteins like grains and beans for complete proteins that include all the amino acids you need.

How can I get started? You can cut your food budget, make healthier meals, and keep your waistline slim — all with one versatile kitchen trick. Use inexpensive canned or dried beans in recipes instead of meat. Beans are rich in fiber, potassium, magnesium, folate, iron, lysine, and zinc. They're a good source of protein and resistant starch, a type of carbohydrate that won't make your blood sugar spike. Diets that include beans reduce LDL cholesterol and cut your risk of heart disease and diabetes. Beans may also help you feel full and control your weight.

Step 3: Lose the fat

Weight loss: lock in your success

There's an old English proverb that says, "Don't dig your grave with your own knife and fork." Let's face it, with nearly one in five deaths in the United States related to obesity, too many people are doing just that.

Carrying a dangerous amount of extra weight is one of the greatest health threats facing people today. It plays a part in serious conditions like heart disease, diabetes, and some cancers. It not only exacts a horrific toll in lives, but it places a crushing burden on our medical system. In the year 2018, experts predict the U.S. will spend $344 billion on obesity-related health care expenses.

This sweeping epidemic is not due to lack of effort or interest. At any given time, anywhere from 50 to 100 million adults are jumping onto the diet bandwagon. And they are spending $20 billion for the ride.

But it's just not working. Why? Because a "diet" almost always has an agenda — usually to sell more diet books or associated products. Ultimately, most diets are all about the three D's — distorted information, deprivation, and, unfortunately, defeat.

To succeed in your quest for a slimmer, healthier you, ditch the fads, the shortcuts, and the magical pills. It's time to take a new approach. Set realistic goals based on your body type, make smart food choices you can live with for the rest of your life, and embrace lifestyle changes that will lock in your success.

Find your happy weight

3 things you didn't know about body fat

Body fat isn't all bad. In fact, fat cells release key hormones and other compounds to help manage important body processes. But too much body fat triggers chemical and physical changes that can cause trouble from your head to your toes.

Fat cells can turn rogue. Normally, fat cells release hormones called adipokines to help your immune system work properly. But when you have too much body fat, your fat cells flood your bloodstream with an overload of adipokines.

These adipokines travel all over your body promoting dangerous, low-grade inflammation and reducing your cells' ability to use insulin properly. That inflammation and insulin resistance raises your risk of diabetes, heart disease, cancer, liver disease, high blood pressure, and stroke. It also ratchets up your odds of metabolic syndrome. This dangerous syndrome combines obesity or being overweight with two of these — high blood sugar, high blood pressure, low HDL cholesterol, or high triglycerides.

Risk of disease increases. Extra fat doesn't just cause life-threatening illnesses. It can affect your daily life as well. For example, every 7 pounds you gain raises your risk of painful gout by 5 percent. Being overweight or obese also raises your risk of these:

- arthritis
- hernias
- kidney stones
- gallstones

- varicose veins
- complications during surgery
- delayed wound healing
- medication dosing errors
- breathing difficulty, including sleep apnea
- higher insurance costs

But losing as little as 5 to 10 pounds can make a positive difference in your chronic health conditions, your risk of disease, and how easily you can do your daily activities. What's more, experts suggest weight loss can also improve arthritis knee pain, your memory, hot flashes, and how well you sleep.

Slim down to put an end to heartburn

Losing weight can improve your heartburn or even make it vanish, and an amazing valve is responsible. This valve, known as the lower esophageal sphincter (LES), separates your stomach from your esophagus, just like a door. It opens long enough to let food in your stomach. Without it, stomach acid would be pushed back into your esophagus as your stomach churns to digest food.

But if you are overweight or obese, extra body fat presses against your stomach. This causes the LES to relax and leak stomach acid into your esophagus, which triggers painful heartburn.

If heartburn interferes with your normal activities every week, you have gastroesophageal reflux disease (GERD). Fortunately, losing weight may help reverse the problem. According to recent studies, more than half of the participants who were overweight or obese improved — or even eliminated — their painful GERD symptoms just by shedding 5 to 10 percent of their body weight.

Polyunsaturated fats fight belly fat. Changing the fats you eat is a smart way to start fighting body fat. A Swedish study found that overeaters who ate more saturated fat gained more belly fat than overeaters who ate less saturated fat. Overeaters who ate more polyunsaturated fats gained more lean muscle and less belly fat — a less-hazardous combination. And it doesn't take much. Add just a half tablespoon of safflower oil to your daily diet. It even works for women over age 50.

Another study found that people who ate more fish rich in omega-3 fats lost more body fat and inches from their waistlines. So limit foods high in saturated fats like fatty cuts of meat, egg yolks, palm or coconut oil, and full-fat dairy. Replace them with foods rich in polyunsaturated or omega-3 fats such as nuts, salmon, sunflower seeds, rainbow trout, sardines, sunflower oil, and peanut butter without added fat.

The key to staying healthy

You have the power to take control of your health. Learning the dangers of being overweight or obese and checking your BMI (body mass index) is a good place to start.

Discover what BMI means for you. BMI helps to determine if you are at a healthy weight for your height. That's important because your risk of weight-related health problems, including heart attacks, diabetes, and stroke, is lower when your BMI falls within the healthy range. The trick is to know what your BMI numbers tell you.

For example, Marilyn Monroe's BMI stayed between 19 and 23 throughout her adult life. Since numbers ranging from 18.5 to 24.9 refer to "normal" weight, she qualified as being at a healthy weight. On the other hand, a BMI under 18.5 means you are underweight like Twiggy was. A BMI of 25 or more means you're overweight, and 30 or higher means you're obese.

To learn your BMI, find your height and weight on the following chart.

Body Mass Index (BMI)

Light shading = overweight
Dark shading = obese

Weight / Height	100	110	120	130	140	150	160	170	180	190	200
5′0″	20	21	23	25	27	29	31	33	35	37	39
5′1″	19	21	23	25	26	28	30	32	34	36	38
5′2″	18	20	22	24	26	27	29	31	33	35	37
5′3″	18	19	21	23	25	27	28	30	32	34	35
5′4″	17	19	21	22	24	26	27	29	31	33	34
5′5″	17	18	20	22	23	25	27	28	30	32	33
5′6″	16	18	19	21	23	24	26	27	29	31	32
5′7″	16	17	19	20	22	23	25	27	28	30	31
5′8″	15	17	18	20	21	23	24	26	27	29	30
5′9″	15	16	18	19	21	22	24	25	27	28	30
5′10″	14	16	17	19	20	22	23	24	26	27	29
5′11″	14	15	17	18	20	21	22	24	25	26	28
6′0″	14	15	16	18	19	20	22	23	24	26	27
6′1″	13	15	16	17	18	20	21	22	24	25	26
6′2″	13	14	15	17	18	19	21	22	23	24	26
6′3″	12	14	15	16	17	19	20	21	22	24	25

If your BMI isn't in the healthy range, notice which weight numbers are healthy for your height.

Cut your odds even more. Just as two heads are better than one, BMI is more valuable when it doesn't work alone. Here's why.

- BMI can give false readings for people with very high amounts of muscle like athletes or weightlifters, or unusually low amounts of muscle that may appear in some overweight women over age 50.
- BMI may be less accurate for people age 65 and up.
- BMI doesn't tell how much dangerous visceral fat you have. Visceral fat increases your risk of disease.

To help solve some of these problems, experts recommend you combine BMI with measuring your waist. This helps you estimate overall fat, as well as visceral fat. For details about this dangerous fat, how to measure for it, and how to get rid of it, keep reading.

Best bets for gaining weight

Being underweight weakens your immune system, raises your risk for osteoporosis and heart problems, and slows wound healing. See your doctor if your BMI is under 18.5, especially if you don't know why your weight is low. To help regain weight, many health professionals recommend these ideas.

- Eat at least five small, frequent meals to feel less full.
- Emphasize high-calorie, high-nutrient foods like lean meats, pasta, whole grains, dairy foods, and produce. Include foods high in unsaturated fats like natural peanut butter, nuts, or avocados.
- Set an alarm to remind yourself to eat.
- Do strength training to build muscle and stimulate your appetite.
- Drink juice, chocolate milk, healthy smoothies, and other beverages after or between meals.
- Keep healthy snacks like trail mix, peanut butter filled celery, or cheese readily available.
- Try larger portions.
- Eat 500 extra calories daily.

Beware a deadly fat lurking in your body

Children and pets may hide when thunder shakes the house, but they have more to fear from lightning than from thunder. A similar problem happens with body fat. People worry about the fat they can see, but the deadliest body fat is the kind you can't see.

Understand fat. Your body can turn extra calories into two kinds of body fat. Most body fat is subcutaneous fat. This sits just under your skin, so it's easy to spot.

Visceral fat dwells deep inside your midsection, where you can't see it. When enough visceral fat accumulates, it pushes subcutaneous fat outward, making your belly bigger. Visceral fat is dangerous because it pumps inflammatory chemicals, fatty acids, and other dangerous compounds into your bloodstream. These cause inflammation and other problems throughout your body, raising your risk of heart disease, diabetes, and other chronic diseases.

You're more likely to have too much visceral fat if most of your body fat is around your midsection and chest (apple shape), rather than around your thighs and buttocks (pear shape). But remember, you can have too much visceral fat even if you don't look overweight. For a better way to measure your risk, measure your waist.

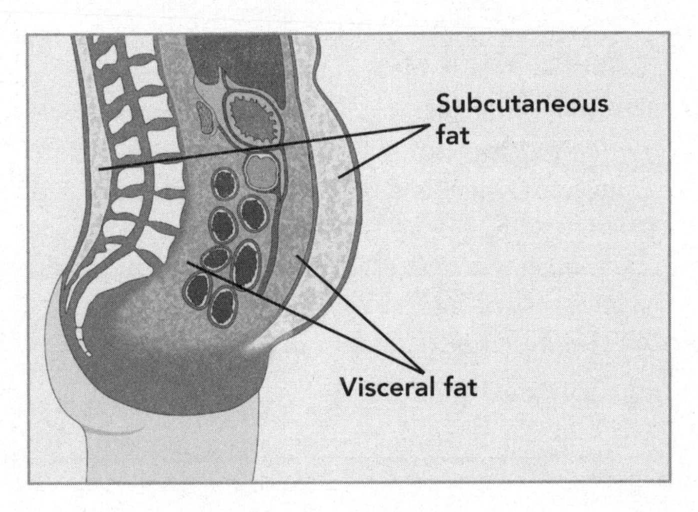

Try a gut check that could save your life. Wrap your measuring tape snugly around your middle so it crosses your belly button and the top of each hipbone. Once you make sure the tape is not tight enough to squeeze your skin, breathe out, and measure. Measure three times, and average the numbers if you get different measurements.

Your results may affect how long you'll live. An analysis of more than 600,000 people made these discoveries.

- Men with waists measuring 43 inches or more faced a higher risk of death than men whose waists were 35 inches or smaller. The added risk from a 43-inch waist was equivalent to cutting three years off the number of years you could expect to live after age 40.
- Women whose waists measured at least 37 inches had a higher risk of death than women with waists under 27 inches. The added risk would be like slashing five years off the number of years you could expect to live after age 40.
- For every 2-inch increase in waist size, risk of an earlier death rose 7 percent in men and 9 percent in women.

To protect yourself, follow the American Heart Association guidelines. They recommend men keep their waistlines below 40 inches and women below 35 inches.

Lose dangerous belly fat. If your waist measurement is too high, many health experts recommend exercising aerobically at least four times each week, and strength training with light weights on the remaining days. But before you start, get your doctor's permission, and see the *Get up and move* section to learn more about these types of activities. Meanwhile, try these daily dining secrets for a flatter tummy.

- Get rid of refined grains. These are grains or grain products whose whole-grain nutrients have been removed. Replace refined-grain breads, cereals, baked goods, and white rice with whole grains like brown rice, oatmeal, whole-grain bread, and wild rice. To learn how to find whole-grain bread, see *Don't be fooled by sneaky bread labels* in the *Quality carbs: put more pep in your step* chapter.
- Eliminate trans fats. You'll find them in packaged foods and fried foods. Read labels to find out which packaged foods have them.

- Eat more soluble fiber from foods like beans, barley, peas, apples, and oatmeal.
- Replace saturated fats with lean protein, and eat plenty of fruits and vegetables.

Surprising cause of obesity your doctor won't tell you about

Starting around age 30, you replace a half pound of muscle with up to a pound of fat every year. Put on enough fat, and you may develop sarcopenic obesity, even with a normal BMI. Sarcopenic obesity means you have too much body fat and not enough muscle. This raises your risk of metabolic syndrome and disability, and it can increase your risk of an earlier death.

When you're dieting, one-fourth of every pound you lose is muscle tissue. Too much muscle loss can lead to serious health problems in older adults.

If your doctor approves, strength exercises or resistance training may help protect you, even without weight loss. But if your doctor recommends losing weight, resistance training helps retain more muscle and burn more fat. To lose even less muscle, some health experts suggest older adults eat the recommended daily amount of protein or more during weight loss. Ask your doctor what you should do.

Outsmart your out-of-control appetite

Gaining weight depends on whether you eat and drink more calories than your body can burn, but that's not all you need to know. The human body is set up to prevent starvation, and that affects you in surprising ways.

Meet your body's savings account. Calories you take in — whether from fats, carbohydrates, or protein — that aren't burned up by your body are stored as body fat. This happens so your body can draw on those reserves if starvation threatens. Unfortunately, this system works almost too well. Your body can store many pounds of fat, and any excess calories you consume transform into body fat within hours. That's why every bite you take matters.

Take the easy path to fewer bites. You need a way you can eat less without feeling hungry all the time. These clever tips will help you feel full sooner.

- Go for protein. Protein is better at making you feel full than fats or carbohydrates, so replace some carbohydrate or fat calories with reduced-calorie protein in most meals and snacks. Good choices include fish, lean meat, skim milk, and other low-fat dairy products.
- Start with a salad. People who began a meal with a 100-calorie salad ate fewer calories at that meal than people who started with 100-calories of garlic bread, according to a British study. To fill up while eating less, choose foods with a high water or fiber content at the beginning of meals or as snacks. If you don't want a salad, try a small cup of soup. Another recent study found that soup lovers had lower body weights, slimmer waistlines, and ate fewer calories than people who didn't eat soup. Other good choices include fruits, vegetables, and beans.
- Eat a little fat. Fat won't help you feel full while eating, but it may keep you from getting hungry between meals.

While you're at it, change habits that can lead you to overeat. For example, eat before you become ravenously hungry. Otherwise, you may be tempted to eat too much.

Similarly, recognize that "cleaning your plate" isn't the only way to prevent food from going to waste. When a portion is too big, stop eating. You don't have to continue eating when you're no longer hungry. Instead, save the extra food for a later meal or snack, or use it as an ingredient in a different dish.

4 ways calorie counts can fool you

A recent headline proclaimed you no longer need to count calories to lose weight. Before you throw away your calorie counter, make sure you know the facts.

- Cooked foods are often assumed to have the same number of calories as the raw version, but cooked foods have more. The reason — it's easier for your body to extract nutrients from foods that are cooked.
- Some foods are digested less completely so the body takes in fewer of the food's calories.
- Processed foods provide more calories than whole foods because processed foods are easier to digest.
- Advertised calorie amounts for restaurant foods and foods with a nutrition label can be off by 20 percent.

But even if calories vary from what you expect, counting calories still helps you lose weight. It keeps you motivated and helps you track how well you're doing. It also helps you catch weight loss problems early and form new, healthy habits.

Powerful secrets of successful losers

Taking steps to eat healthier and eat less is a great idea, but don't stop there. Hedge your bets with terrific tools that have already helped others lose weight and keep it off.

Estimate your daily goal. Before starting any weight loss plan, check with your doctor to make sure you can lose weight safely, and confirm you've set the best weight goal.

On average, doctors recommend cutting 500 to 1,000 calories a day so you can lose 1 to 2 pounds a week. But this method doesn't tell you how many calories you should eat to maintain your new weight once you reach your goal. This varies depending on how active you are. So plan for:

- 12 calories per pound of body weight if you're sedentary.
- 15 calories per pound if you get 30 minutes or more of moderate to intense exercise daily.
- 13 or 14 per pound if you fall somewhere in between.

To calculate your daily calorie goal, multiply your weight goal by calories per pound of body weight. For example, if you're sedentary and hope to lose enough weight to reach 125 pounds, you multiply 125 by 12 for a total of 1,500 calories.

Just remember, doctors recommend women never take in less than 1,200 calories a day and men should not consume less than 1,500 calories daily unless the diet is medically supervised. So set your calorie goal no lower than these numbers. Diets below these calorie levels often fail, and are unlikely to supply enough nutrients to keep you healthy. Diets under 1,100 calories may also cause hair loss, fatigue, dizziness, or gallstones.

Lose twice the weight with tracking. A study in the *American Journal of Preventive Medicine* found that people who kept complete daily food diaries lost twice as much weight as people who didn't. In contrast, some people who have lost weight, but stopped counting calories, report that they began regaining weight. So for best results, keep a food diary, and track your calories.

To start your own food diary, record everything you eat and drink in a paper journal, online diary, cellphone notepad program, or smartphone app. Include how much of each item you ate or drank, calories for each item if available, and the time of day. You can also include how hungry you were, your mood, and where you ate.

Determine how much food you are eating by checking the serving size on product labels, or using measuring cups, measuring spoons, or a food scale before you eat.

You also need to translate servings into calories. If you have a smartphone, a free app such as Calorie Counter may provide calorie counts for foods you record while on the go. You may also find calorie counts on package labels. If calorie counts aren't readily available, tally them when you get home. To find out how many calories are in a food, use a reference book you buy or borrow from the library, or check a website such as *nutrition-data.self.com* or Food-A-Pedia from *www.supertracker.usda.gov*.

Review your diary regularly to uncover:

- whether you exceeded your daily calorie goal.
- where you can cut back with the least discomfort.
- opportunities to shift more of your planned calories to foods you like.
- incidents when you ate more calories than you thought.
- what triggers eating too many calories.
- which foods you get the most calories from.
- whether changes you make are effective.

Check your progress. People who weighed themselves daily or weekly lost more weight than people who only stepped on the scales once a month, a study found. And the more weight people needed to lose, the better frequent weigh-ins worked. Other studies show that people who weigh themselves more often also regain less weight. Frequent weighing helps keep small weight gains from turning into large ones.

Little-known crash-dieting danger

Obesity raises your odds of painful gallstones. But losing weight too quickly or losing and regaining can raise your risk, too. Women who have experienced gallstone pain say it can be worse than childbirth. To help protect yourself, remember these important points.

- People who lose more than 3 pounds each week face a higher gallstone danger. Choose a weight loss plan that helps you shed 2 pounds or less each week.

- Dieters on a 500-calorie diet were three times as likely to develop gallstones as people on a 1,200- to 1,500-calorie diet, a Swedish study found. Why? During rapid weight loss, your body produces more cholesterol. If too much cholesterol lingers in your gallbladder, gallstones are more likely to form. To help prevent that, avoid crash diets with limits of 800 calories or less a day.
- Each time you lose weight and regain it, you're yo-yo dieting or weight cycling. The more weight you lose and the more often you weight cycle, the higher your risk of gallstones.

9 nutritious snacks to control hunger between meals

Don't be tempted by high-calorie soft drinks, candy bars, or chips when you hit that mid-afternoon slump. For less than 200 calories, you can enjoy one of these satisfying substitutes.

- 1 cup of black bean soup
- large orange and a half cup of low-fat vanilla yogurt
- 3 cups of air-popped popcorn with hot sauce or Italian spices
- single serve instant oatmeal with fresh or frozen blueberries
- 4 raw figs
- 8 ounces of low-fat chocolate milk
- 1 cup of puffed rice cereal with skim milk and cinnamon
- large apple with a 1-ounce slice of low-fat cheddar cheese
- 2 cups of celery strips, cauliflower, sliced summer squash, or other raw vegetables with a half cup of salsa, three tablespoons of hummus, or three tablespoons of reduced-fat Italian dressing

Promising new way to measure body fat

Move over BMI. A new body fat measurement called A Body Shape Index (ABSI) may be better at predicting your risk of an early death. Unlike BMI, ABSI includes your waist measurement and age in its calculations. Although more research is needed to confirm that ABSI is best, you can try it today if you have access to the Web. Search for "ABSI calculator," or visit *www-ce.ccny.cuny.edu/nir/sw/absi-calculator.html.*

To see what your ABSI results mean, check "Relative risk from ABSI." Numbers below one mean your risk of an early death is below average. Numbers above one mean danger. For example, a 1.2 means your odds of an early death are 20 percent higher than average. Just remember, exercise and a healthier diet can still help you lower that risk.

Create a diet plan that works for you

Actor Mark Wahlberg lost 60 pounds in just four months for a starring role in a movie, but the drastic diet made him so miserable he said he would never do it again. Since misery isn't your goal either, choose a nourishing diet plan you can live with — or create your own.

Learn from the experts. You've probably heard about low-fat diets, low-carbohydrate diets, high-protein diets, and low- or no-protein diets. Many studies have compared diets like these, which contain various mixes of fat, carbohydrates, and protein. But in their recent article in the *Journal of the American Medical Association*, researchers Dr. Sherry Pagoto and Dr. Bradley Appelhans point out three things.

- Studies find that no one diet is consistently much better at weight loss than the others.
- When one diet beats other diets in a study, the difference is less than 5 pounds.

- The one consistent finding from studies is this — the longer people can stick with a diet, the better their results.

So when you choose a diet or design your own, aim for one you can easily follow every day for a long time. Also, choose a diet that supplies enough nutrients, so you won't be plagued by side effects from a nutritional deficiency. Experts generally recommend a diet containing 45 to 65 percent carbohydrates, 10 to 35 percent protein, and 20 to 35 percent fat. But if that sounds too complicated, choose your calorie goal, and select a diet with a mix of foods similar to this chart.

Calories	Vegetables	Fruits	Grains	Dairy	Protein	Oils	Solid fats & added sugars	Sodium
1,600	2 cups	1 1/2 cups	5 oz.	3 cups	5 oz.	5 tsp.	120 calories	2,300 mg (1 tsp.)
1,800	2 1/2 cups	1 1/2 cups	6 oz.	3 cups	5 oz.	5 tsp.	160 calories	2,300 mg (1 tsp.)
2,000	2 1/2 cups	2 cups	6 oz.	3 cups	5 1/2 oz.	6 tsp.	260 calories	2,300 mg (1 tsp.)
2,200	3 cups	2 cups	7 oz.	3 cups	6 oz.	6 tsp.	270 calories	2,300 mg (1 tsp.)
2,400	3 cups	2 cups	8 oz.	3 cups	6 1/2 oz.	7 tsp.	330 calories	2,300 mg (1 tsp.)
2,600	3 1/2 cups	2 cups	9 oz.	3 cups	6 1/2 oz.	8 tsp.	360 calories	2,300 mg (1 tsp.)
2,800	3 1/2 cups	2 1/2 cups	10 oz.	3 cups	7 oz.	8 tsp.	400 calories	2,300 mg (1 tsp.)
3,000	4 cups	2 1/2 cups	10 oz.	3 cups	7 oz.	10 tsp.	460 calories	2,300 mg (1 tsp.)
3,200	4 cups	2 1/2 cups	10 oz.	3 cups	7 oz.	11 tsp.	600 calories	2,300 mg (1 tsp.)

Build on your success. To eat a well-rounded diet, also plan your meals around these tips.

- Choose low-fat or nonfat dairy and lean cuts of meat and poultry.
- Include fish twice a week, and use beans, nuts, peas, or seeds as your protein from time to time.
- Eat more whole grains than refined grains.
- Enjoy a mix of vegetables each week, including red or orange vegetables, dark green vegetables, starchy vegetables, and beans or peas.
- Consume more solid fruits than fruit juices.
- Read food labels to accurately follow your diet. Labels can help you determine how many ounces of grain you're eating or whether a food is truly low in fat, calories, added sugars, saturated fats, or other ingredients. For more information about food labels, see *New food label cuts the confusion* in the *Food smarts: heroes to zeroes* chapter.
- Check calorie and fat content of drinks, toppings, spreads, and sauces.

Ditch the troublemakers. Say goodbye to junk food and try new, interesting recipes, ingredients, and restaurant offerings in place of high-calorie foods. Choose items that are tasty and low-calorie — and only continue to buy or make the ones you look forward to eating.

Peel away pounds without feeling deprived

"Fruits and vegetables won't help you lose weight," the headlines howled. But the same study that led to those headlines also hints at how eating produce can still be a great way to slim down.

Good news if you struggle with obesity

Obesity is now officially recognized as a disease by the American Medical Association. In 2013, the American Heart Association also recommended doctors treat obesity as a disease. This could mean more help for people who struggle with obesity.

In the past, one-third of obese people reported that doctors never mentioned their weight. Now, more doctors may counsel patients about obesity and offer treatment. The American Medical Association and the American Heart Association also hope insurance companies will increase reimbursement for weight loss treatments.

If you're obese, don't wait for your doctor to talk about weight loss. Ask your insurer what obesity coverage and programs you qualify for and request details about costs and coverage rules. For example, Medicare participants may qualify for intensive behavioral counseling for obesity, including personalized advice and obesity-fighting techniques. Private health insurance companies may offer similar options.

Make friends with fruits and veggies. "Unfortunately, it seems that if we just get people to eat more fruits and vegetables without also taking explicit steps to reduce total food intake, lower weights are not achieved," says study author David B. Allison, an associate dean at the University of Alabama at Birmingham.

In other words, if you normally eat 2,000 calories a day, and start eating an extra 300 calories of fruits and vegetables, your diet increases to 2,300 calories a day, and you won't lose weight. But another study shows vegetables and fruit can still help.

This study compared meat-eaters to several groups including:

- strict vegetarians.
- people who only ate meat occasionally.

- those vegetarians who eat dairy foods and eggs.
- vegetarians who also ate fish.

Meat eaters had the highest BMI and were the most likely to be obese. Occasional meat eaters and fish-eating vegetarians had lower BMIs. Strict vegetarians had the lowest BMIs and the lowest odds of obesity.

So the best way to save both money and calories may be this. Substitute vegetables and fruits for part of the meat. For a tasty way to start, take a tip from restaurant chefs.

Learn secrets from top chefs. Chefs at many high-end restaurants mix mushrooms into their hamburger meat and other meat dishes. To try this at home, lightly sauté a pound of finely minced white button mushrooms in 2 tablespoons of canola oil. Season to taste and cook until the moisture has evaporated. You can add the cooked mushroom mixture to raw, ground meat for hamburgers, or cook the meat in a skillet with the sautéed mushrooms to use in tacos, lasagna, or other favorites.

Your dishes will taste terrific, but you'll eat less meat, which means fewer calories. Don't want to use mushrooms? Substitute beans for half the meat in your recipe, or stretch the recipe with three-fourths cup of pureed veggies per pound of meat.

Also, try replacing meat entrees like fried chicken with meat-vegetable dishes like chicken stir-fry with vegetables. You can even experiment with vegetarian dishes like bean burritos, pineapple pizza, or a tomato-avocado sandwich.

Sneaky diet foods that add pounds

You may think fat-free cookies are helping you lose weight, but don't be fooled. Foods touted as fat free, reduced fat, or low fat may not contain much less fat than the originals. What's more, they may make up the calories with added sugar or other ingredients. Before you bite, check the food's label, or look up the nutrition information online. Note the serving size and calorie count to see if you'll be eating more calories than you expect. Do the same for other diet food traps like these.

- fast food salads or salad kits
- gluten-free foods
- vitamin waters, sports drinks, and many other bottled drinks
- low-sugar foods

Trade problem diet foods for edibles that may help with weight loss. For example, low-calorie foods that contain chili peppers or red pepper may help burn a few extra calories, reduce your appetite, and fight abdominal fat. And eating a small handful of tree nuts, such as walnuts, almonds, and Brazil nuts, once a week has been linked to lower odds of obesity. Tree nuts are good sources of fiber and protein, which help you feel full.

Is MSG a secret cause of weight gain?

Monosodium glutamate (MSG), a flavor enhancer added to many foods, could literally be weighing you down. A recent study found that animals given MSG gained more weight than animals not getting this additive. But studies with people reveal a different story.

Research in the *British Journal of Nutrition* did not find a connection between the MSG people ate and their weight. Yet another study reported that people who ate the most MSG every day were more likely to be overweight than people who ate the least, even though they both consumed the same amount of calories. Clearly, additional research is needed to find out whether MSG can affect your weight.

Meanwhile, if you are concerned about possible weight gain from MSG, reduce the amount in your daily diet. Check for MSG in the ingredient labels of foods before you buy, and ask about the MSG content in restaurant foods before you order.

Diet drinks: weight loss wonder or diet blunder?

Enjoy that mid-afternoon Snickers bar with a low-calorie Diet Coke instead of regular Coke, and you will cut calories. But recent research suggests you may be sabotaging your weight loss plan.

Researchers from Johns Hopkins University studied diet beverages and calorie consumption in adults. Here's what they found.

- Among overweight and obese adults, diet beverage drinkers took in more calories from food than people who drank sugar-sweetened beverages. The researchers suspect they may eat extra food to make up for the missing calories. Artificial sweeteners might also increase your appetite or affect the "sweet sensors" in your brain, decreasing the satisfaction you get from eating something sweet. If you want to use diet drinks to lose weight, the study authors suggest you track how many calories you eat and drink, and make sure you're reducing your total calorie intake.
- Among people who weren't overweight or obese, diet beverage drinkers took in fewer total calories a day than people who drank sugar-sweetened beverages. So if your weight is normal, switching from sugar-sweetened beverages to diet drinks may help you prevent weight gain.

Diet drinks may affect more than just your weight. Some studies suggest they may also raise your risk of diabetes, heart attacks, and strokes. Sugar-sweetened beverages have also been linked to bigger waistlines and elevated blood sugar and triglyceride levels, which can increase your risk for diabetes or heart disease.

That's why some experts suggest you limit or eliminate both sugar-sweetened beverages and diet drinks. Instead, emphasize better choices like water, sparkling water, and unsweetened coffee or tea.

Tactics to win the weight-loss war

Fat-burning secrets for easier weight loss

Americans spend more than $20 billion a year trying to lose weight, yet more than two-thirds of U.S. adults are overweight. Learn more about how your body manages calories, so you can find the best ways to lose weight without breaking the bank.

Three ways to burn calories. These things determine the number of calories you burn each day:

- Basal metabolic rate (BMR). Your body needs energy to breathe, make your heart beat, and perform all the other processes that keep you going. The total calories you burn to fuel these involuntary activities is your BMR. This accounts for up to 70 percent of the calories you burn each day. BMR drops about 5 percent with each passing decade, which means you burn fewer calories as you age.
- Thermogenesis. This is the energy you use to digest food, absorb nutrients, and store excess calories as body fat. Up to 10 percent of calories you burn go to thermogenesis.
- Exercise. Physical activity accounts for the remaining calories you burn. Increasing your daily activities helps you burn more calories, but if you want to raise your BMR, exercise to build more muscle. Muscle tissue burns more calories than fat.

Altogether, this means you have two ways to fend off extra pounds — eat less and exercise more. Once you burn more calories than you take in, you start losing weight. If you're overweight or obese, that's also when you begin getting healthier. Just be sure to get your doctor's permission before starting an exercise program.

Surprising exercise secrets. Think twice before you try killer workouts or avoid exercise to tame your appetite. Research suggests better ways to go.

- Start small and work up to a higher intensity. Overweight or obese women who only did light or moderate aerobic exercise still lost weight, decreased body fat, and added muscle, a recent study found. What's more, a Danish study found that men who exercised half an hour daily for 12 weeks lost at least as much weight as men who exercised a full hour. The half-hour group was more likely to exercise every day and reported feeling more energetic and motivated to exercise.

- Exercise to control your hunger. Appetite is suppressed right after a workout. For several hours, you also fill up more quickly and are less hungry between meals. Just eat sensibly after working out. Don't reward yourself with a high-calorie treat, or you may consume more calories than your exercise burned.

- Alternate aerobic with resistance exercises. When you diet without exercising, the pounds you lose include both fat and muscle tissue. People who add exercise to a reduced-calorie diet lose less muscle and more fat. They also regain less weight. To build more muscle and burn more calories, alternate the days you do aerobic exercise with days of resistance exercise, or strength training, with light weights. Resistance training may help burn 100 extra calories — or more — every day.

What to do if you're hungry all the time

Hungry? Even after meals? You could have leptin resistance. This condition is named for leptin, a hormone your fat cells produce to tell you when you've had enough food. Some overweight people create too much leptin. Over time, this leads to the nearly constant hunger of leptin resistance.

Fortunately, you can take steps to prevent this, even before you begin losing weight. Research suggests regular exercise and good sleep habits can help prevent leptin resistance. Losing weight will help even more.

Restaurant survival guide

Dining out adds 200 extra calories to your daily total, a recent study found. You'd get nearly the same number of calories from a Hershey's Milk Chocolate Bar. But don't stop eating out. Use these clever tricks to find low-calorie items hidden in the restaurant menu.

- Call ahead or check the restaurant's nutrition information on its website to find healthy, low-calorie dishes. Before you try to estimate calories by looking at the dish or its menu description, consider this. A recent study found that people underestimated the calorie content of restaurant food by at least 175 calories, and some underestimate by 500 calories. The higher the calories in a meal, the more people underestimate. If you can't check calories, order from the low-calorie or heart-healthy menu, or ask your server which low-calorie dishes are the best.
- Order water, unsweetened tea, fat-free or low-fat milk, or other drinks without added sugars.

- Ask for whole-wheat bread if you order a sandwich.
- Avoid the all-you-can-eat buffet. Order from the menu instead.
- Beware the super-size bargain. Think twice before you upgrade to the larger portion for a lower price per serving. You may get a good deal, but you'll get too many calories if you eat it all at once. Only consider deals like these if you share with another person or take home the extra food for another meal. Sharing and doggy bags are also a good way to keep from eating regular-size portions that are too high in calories.
- Ask for salad dressing on the side so you can choose how much to use. Watch out for salad saboteurs including high-fat dressings, candied nuts, and meats that are breaded or drowning in sauce. Also, avoid salads where the vegetables and fruit are outnumbered by meats, cheeses, mayo, croutons, and other ingredients high in saturated fats or calories.
- Choose main dishes that include vegetables and grains, such as stir fries, red beans and rice, kebobs, or pasta with a tomato sauce.
- Avoid fried dishes, and order options that are grilled, broiled, or steamed.
- Opt for the small, medium, or appetizer size if the entree, drink, or side dish comes in more than one size.
- Order all sauces on the side.
- Ask for substitutions. For example, substitute rice pilaf for a side of fries, or marinara sauce for Alfredo sauce.
- Never add butter or salt to foods.
- Enjoy fresh fruit for dessert.

Flatten your belly naturally

You can melt away belly fat in just five minutes each morning — and it doesn't involve doing sit-ups.

Grab a bowl. Researchers studying people ages 60 to 80 made a fascinating discovery. The more fiber the study participants ate, the less body fat and belly fat they had, especially if a lot of their fiber came from breakfast cereal. In fact, those who got more fiber from breakfast cereal had significantly less belly fat than everyone else in the study.

Although the researchers weren't sure why cereal fiber helped, many studies suggest fiber reduces hunger and makes you feel full longer. That means it will be easier to eat less at your next meal.

Experts recommend slowly working up to three servings of whole grains a day. Examples of a serving include a cup of ready-to-eat, whole-grain cereal or a half cup of hot, whole-grain cereal. Those servings come with a sweet payoff. Studies show the more whole grains and grain fiber people eat:

- the less visceral belly fat they have.
- the lower their BMI and weight.
- the smaller their waists.
- the lower their risk of gaining weight.

What's more, a study of obese dieters who ate whole grains found they lost more belly fat in three months than obese dieters who only ate refined grains.

Play it safe. If you aren't getting much fiber, take five minutes to enjoy a bowl of hot or cold whole-grain cereal every morning. Not only can whole-grain cereal help fight belly fat, it's also a good way to gradually increase your fiber and whole-grain intake.

People who add too much fiber too quickly may experience diarrhea, gas, bloating, and stomach pain. So add fiber gradually in small amounts, and cut back if you run into trouble.

Why fast weight-loss strategies backfire

Cutting calories to shed pounds is the best way to lose weight, but if you cut too much, your body's anti-starvation defenses kick in. That may explain why a recent University of Illinois study revealed that women who skip meals lose less weight than women who don't.

Experts aren't sure whether skipping a meal leads to overeating later, or whether something else about missing meals makes weight loss tougher. But either way, skipping meals won't help you lose more weight.

Crash dieting seems like a good alternative, but rapid weight loss melts away muscle tissue as well as fat. Since muscle burns more calories, every pound you lose reduces your body's ability to burn calories, a preliminary study suggests. If future research backs up this study, it could explain why losing weight seems to get increasingly harder during a crash diet, but gaining it all back becomes easier and easier.

Easy ways to slash 100 extra calories every day

Eat one extra pat of butter on your baked potato and four extra Ritz crackers with your salad, and you'll add 100 calories to your day. Portion sizes creep up so subtly you don't even realize you're eating more. Unfortunately, experts warn that as little as 100 extra calories a day can lead to a 10-pound weight gain every year.

Take control of portion sizes. When you can't bring your own food or measure what you eat, use this handy chart to help estimate portion sizes to avoid overeating.

Food	Equivalent measure
1 cup of chopped or cut raw fruits or vegetables	a woman's fist (from wrist to knuckles) or a baseball
1/4 cup of dried fruit	a golf ball or small handful
medium apple or orange	a tennis ball
3 oz. serving of meat or poultry	the palm of your hand or a deck of cards
3 oz. serving of fish	a checkbook
1 1/2 to 2 oz. cheese	4 dice
1/2 cup steamed or cooked rice	a cupcake wrapper
1/2 cup cooked pasta or mashed potatoes	a rounded handful or tennis ball
1/3 cup of pretzels or chips	a level handful
1 oz. of nuts	a handful
2 tbsp. of peanut butter	a golf or ping pong ball
1-oz. or 1 tbsp. serving of butter, salad dressing, sour cream, or cream cheese	your thumb
1 tsp. of margarine, oil, butter, or sugar	your thumb tip

Guard against sneaky pounds. These tips can help you keep your weight under control.

- Check the calories and serving size on the label before eating or preparing a food. Serving sizes are smaller than you think. Avoid eating directly from the package, and measure out the appropriate serving instead of estimating the right size.

- Check daily to see if you're eating the right amount of calories to lose weight. To learn how to count the calories you eat and calculate a good calorie goal for weight loss, see the *Find your happy weight* chapter.

- Freeze single-servings of perishable food when you buy or cook in bulk. Otherwise, you may overeat to finish the food before it goes bad.
- Repackage nonperishable foods into single serving packages.
- Don't mix eating with other activities like watching television, reading, or surfing the Web.
- Prevent extra calories from vending machines, restaurants, and convenience stores when traveling or on the go. Bring your own low-calorie snacks, drinks, and meals. Repackage them into the right portion size, and use a cooler for perishable items if a refrigerator isn't available.

Beef up your willpower

Eating too much is easy when food is all around you, so try mindful eating — paying closer attention to what you eat and how much you eat. Here's how it can work for you.

- Stay out of your kitchen between meals if seeing food makes you want to eat. And don't store treats in tabletop candy dishes or on countertops.
- Eating from a plate that's the same color as your food can encourage you to eat more, one study found. Serve the food on a plate that's a dramatically different color — like cream-colored fettuccine Alfredo on a red plate.
- Dine like a restaurant reviewer. Savor your food long enough to describe how it looks on your plate, how it tastes, its texture, and how it compares to similar dishes. Also, notice how many bites it takes to fill you up.

5 tactics to beat emotional eating

You've had a horrible day, so you plunge into a hot fudge sundae to ease your stress. To stop bingeing on comfort food and get back on track, try these techniques.

Double-check your appetite. Before you eat, ask yourself if you are really hungry — or just bored, tired, frustrated, or stressed.

Treat negative thoughts as clues. Replace self-defeating thoughts like "I've failed" or "Trying to lose weight is too hard" with questions like "What triggered my eating?" and "How can I change this behavior?" You'll find answers by keeping a detailed diary of the foods you ate and your emotional and physical state when you began eating. This can help you identify what triggers stressful eating. With that knowledge, you can find ways to manage those triggers.

Clear your path to success. Make sure you get enough sleep and exercise, and check your stress levels regularly. Take additional steps to manage stress if it's affecting your eating habits.

Review your options. Compare what you can have now to the bigger rewards you could get later. For example, you might ask yourself "Would I rather have a treat right now or fit into smaller pants when I go to my high school reunion?"

Find another form of comfort. Distract yourself from eating with these proven suggestions.

- Brush your teeth or drink a tall glass of water.
- Watch a movie, work out, or take a long walk.
- Play a card game, call a friend, listen to music, or do something you enjoyed during childhood, such as puzzles.

- Listen to a favorite song or comedy routine, read a riveting short story, write a quick entry in your weight-loss journal, or indulge in a few minutes of your favorite hobby.
- Enjoy a stress-reducing activity, such as meditating or deep breathing. If you can't do that, drink black tea or chew sugarless gum. Studies suggest these two things reduce your levels of cortisol, the hormone associated with stress.

Don't let little mishaps sabotage your diet

You won't believe what a recent study of NFL football fans discovered. When their favorite team lost on Sunday, football fans took in more calories and saturated fat than usual on Monday to help them cope with defeat. But fans of winning teams actually cut back on saturated fat and calories on the day after the game. Winning actually boosted their self-control.

Regardless of which sport you love and how well your favorite team does, you can prevent comfort eating after your team loses. Study participants quickly returned to their usual eating habits if they took a few minutes after the game to write down what was most important to them in life. The next time your team loses, give this a try. You have nothing to lose but pounds.

Future 'magic' pill may double weight loss

Lose weight faster, slim your waistline, and strip away dangerous visceral fat. You might expect this kind of success from a weight-loss drug, but researchers have recently shown you can get these results from a more surprising source — the friendly bacteria living in your gut.

Probiotics are the good bacteria that benefit your health. These probiotics not only perform tasks that keep you healthy, they also battle harmful bacteria that could make you sick. In fact, experts suggest some health problems get their start when antibiotics or other disruptions leave you with more bad bacteria than good ones.

Fortunately, you can eat probiotic foods or take probiotic supplements that contain millions of living probiotics similar to the ones in your gut. Many kinds of probiotics exist, but research suggests some members of the *Lactobacillus* family may help reduce cravings and the hormones that promote fat storage. And that may not be all probiotics can do.

Canadian women who took a special probiotic called *Lactobacillus rhamnosus CGMCC1.3724* lost twice as much weight as women who didn't get the probiotic, even though both groups followed the same diet. What's more, probiotic takers also reduced their levels of intestinal bacteria linked with obesity. They even ended up with less body fat and lower levels of the appetite regulating hormone, leptin. Just remember — one of the Canadian researchers says you might need to take probiotics like this one with a low-fat, fiber-rich diet for best results.

Meanwhile, Japanese study participants who ate a yogurt containing *Lactobacillus gasseri SBT2055 (LG2055)* not only reduced their body fat, they also cut their waist size and BMI and got rid of dangerous visceral fat.

Unfortunately, the specialty probiotics used in these studies are not available in the United States, but they could turn up in supplements or foods at any time. Keep an eye out for them at your supermarket and drugstore.

Unleash your brain's natural appetite suppressors

Eat foods rich in fermentable fiber, and your body may make its own appetite suppressors, according to new research. You'll find fermentable fiber in fruits, vegetables, barley, and oats. You can't digest fermentable fibers, so bacteria in your colon ferment them. That triggers the release of acetate, an appetite-squelching short-chain fatty acid.

A recent animal study suggests acetate travels to your brain where it raises acetate levels in your hypothalamus, the area of your brain that controls hunger. The resulting chain reaction activates appetite-suppressing neurons.

Eating fermentable fibers may also produce other short-chain fatty acids like butyrate and propionate. New animal research from Europe suggests your intestines use these small fat molecules to produce glucose, which travels through your bloodstream to your liver's portal vein. When glucose arrives, nearby nerves send a message to your brain that helps reduce hunger, cuts glucose production, and burns more calories when you're at rest.

4 fat-blasting sleep habits you can start tonight

How much sleep you get can affect your weight. While lack of sleep could lead to extra eating, scientists now say other sleep-related habits can affect your weight, too. Even worse, they do it the sneaky way — by fouling up your body clock and the hormones that control appetite. That's why the latest research offers more powerful and precise ways to slumber your way to slim.

Adjust your night light. Experts suspect extra light from clock radios, televisions, computers, streetlights, or other sources may affect the production of melatonin, a hormone that helps you sleep. The more light in your bedroom at night, the higher your odds of obesity, suggests a British study. Although the researchers say they can't guarantee a darker room will keep you slim, it's still worth trying. Experiment with simple changes like dimming or turning off night lights and electronics, using blackout curtains or a sleep mask, and turning off unnecessary lights.

Cling to a consistent schedule. Studies suggest people who keep to the same bedtime every night and wake at the same time have less body fat and lower odds of obesity. If you usually set your own sleep schedule, always go to bed within 15 minutes of your normal bedtime and wake within 15 minutes of your regular waking time. If you must set your sleep schedule by your work hours or some other factor beyond your control, one expert suggests:

- scheduling more time in bright light during the morning and less at night to fall asleep earlier.
- getting most of your bright light during afternoon and evening if you fall asleep too early.

Skip nine-hour nights. Averaging more than 8 1/2 hours of sleep each night is linked with more body fat, a recent study found. Authorities suggest you get 6 1/2 to 8 1/2 hours each night to fend off fat.

Keep your cool. Research finds that poor sleep quality means more body fat. So if you're lying awake in bed or sleeping poorly, experts think that may affect hormones associated with eating. To help avoid that, adopt habits like keeping your bedroom comfortably cool and quiet, as well as making sure you don't use the bedroom for watching television, work, or any stressful activity. For more "sleep tight" strategies, see the *Sleep right to save your life* chapter.

Simple way to give your metabolism a boost

People who enjoy bright outdoor light in the morning have a lower body mass index (BMI) than people who are exposed to bright light later, a Northwestern University study reports. Experts suspect this bright light affects your body clock in ways that influence your metabolism and your weight.

To put this to work for you, aim for 20 minutes of bright light every morning, and settle for dimmer light the rest of the day. Even on cloudy days, outdoor light measures over 1,000 on a scale of brightness, while indoor lighting usually rates 300 or less. So your best bet is to spend 20 minutes outside to make sure you get light that is bright enough.

7 proven ways to resist temptation

The best way to succeed at losing weight is to plan for failure. After all, holidays, grocery store freebies, and other temptations are bound to crop up. Experts say you're more likely to stick to your diet if you plan for each one. Start with proven ideas like these.

Avoid supermarket impulse buys. Plan every meal and snack for the upcoming week, and be sure each one meets your weight-loss goals. Make a grocery list so you are less prone to pick up high-calorie items on a whim.

Use coupons with caution. A study of coupons from six retail chains found that most of the coupons offer discounts for high-calorie or unhealthy products. Only use coupons for foods that fit your calorie goals.

Practice polite refusal. Check your calendar for upcoming social occasions, shared meals, or meetings where you'll be offered food you shouldn't eat. Plan what to say to graciously and diplomatically turn down the offer.

Bring your own. Don't get ambushed by a snack attack during an afternoon slump. Instead of raiding vending machines or grabbing a high-calorie snack, have a tasty, low-calorie snack already prepared. To make sure diet-friendly food is available at parties or family gatherings, offer to bring a dish or appetizer.

Plan for evenings out. Researchers found that people were more likely to blow their diets when going out with friends at night. Even if they never pressure you, just being with them can encourage poor choices. Exposure to tempting foods can also be a problem. Before you go out, plan how you'll resist these temptations.

Stack the odds in your favor. A rough morning can make temptation tough to resist for the rest of the day. Plan several quick ways to recharge or reduce stress — like taking a walk or listening to your favorite music.

Removing sources of temptation can help, too. For example, clear your kitchen of foods that aren't diet friendly, and replace them with appetizing alternatives. If your family insists on problem foods, reserve a shelf in your refrigerator and pantry for your low-calorie favorites.

Prepare for unexpected temptation. When you run into a temptation you didn't plan for, change the subject, turn away, or distract yourself as quickly as possible. According to researchers, the more time you spend mulling over your options, the more likely you are to give in.

Breakfast: waist slenderizer or waste of time?

Recent research from the University of Alabama at Birmingham (UAB) seems to suggest eating breakfast regularly won't help you lose weight. But before you start skipping breakfast, get both sides of the story.

The case against breakfast. In an early examination of breakfast research on obesity, UAB researchers found that many of the previous studies on eating or skipping breakfast were either biased or failed to prove the value of breakfast in weight loss. As a result, they concluded too little evidence was available to prove that eating breakfast helps fight obesity.

In more recent research, scientists only found two studies that tested whether regularly eating or skipping breakfast affects weight. Neither study found a connection, but one study suggested results depend on your usual breakfast habits.

The latest evidence. The most recent research may offer more specific information about breakfast. For example, a University of Missouri study shows that eating breakfast may help reduce food cravings, especially if the meal is high in protein.

And since your body is naturally better at burning calories in the morning, eating more of your calories then may not be a bad idea. In fact, one study of overweight and obese women with metabolic syndrome put this to the test.

The researchers compared eating a 700-calorie breakfast followed by a smaller lunch and dinner to eating a 200-calorie breakfast followed by larger meals. Women who ate a 700-calorie breakfast lost more weight and more waistline inches than women who ate the 200-calorie breakfast. The high-calorie breakfast eaters also felt full longer.

Finally, a recent British study suggests breakfast may also help you be more active in the morning, keep better control over your blood sugar, and burn a few extra calories. So even if you don't eat when you roll out of bed, consider eating a midmorning snack.

Dodge dieting dangers

Secret to finding the perfect diet

Every diet claims to be the best choice for weight loss. To find the true champion, Canadian researchers compared popular diets to see which one peeled off the most pounds in a year. At first, a few diets seemed to pull ahead of the pack. Yet, by 12 months, low-fat and low-carbohydrate diets barely performed better than more balanced diets.

Why? Nearly every diet followed the same pattern. People lost weight during the first six months, but regained several pounds by year's end. The researchers concluded the ideal diet is the one you can stick with the longest.

Pick your type. To help you choose, consider the foods you love. You can select a balanced diet that's low in carbohydrates, fat, or calories.

- Balanced diets allow between 45 and 65 percent of your calories to come from carbohydrates, 10 to 35 percent from protein, and 20 to 35 percent from fats. The Weight Watchers and Zone diets fall into this category.
- Low-carbohydrate diets usually limit carbohydrates to no more than 45 percent of calories, and some diets also allow large amounts of calories from protein. Reducing carbohydrates may force your body to burn fat for energy instead of carbohydrates. When a low-carbohydrate diet is also high in protein, the added protein may help prevent hunger. Examples of low-carbohydrate diets include the Atkins, Paleo, and South Beach diets.

- Low-fat diets, like the Ornish and TLC diets, usually limit fat to 20 percent of calories or less.
- Low- or very-low-calorie diets, such as the Slim-Fast diet, may restrict calories to levels below amounts considered safe for most adults.

Compare costs. Prepackaged programs like Jenny Craig can cost around $2,500 a year, and Weight Watchers may cost up to $377. Some diets require you to buy special products, expensive ingredients, or books. Before you choose a diet, tally its monthly costs.

Ask the right questions. The more closely a diet matches your lifestyle, schedule, and habits, the easier it will be to stick with. If you consider a particular diet, get answers to these questions before you try it.

- Does the diet require more work and time than you put into meals and snacks now?
- Will you diet alone, with a partner, or with a support group? Can dieting with other people provide the right mix of encouragement and accountability to help you stick with the diet, or will you end up frustrated?
- Can you still eat out?
- Will the diet help you maintain your goal weight after you finish shedding pounds?
- How restrictive is the diet?
- How much convenience will you give up?
- Will you be hungry often, or does the diet help prevent hunger?
- Does the diet include appetizing foods or opportunities to find new recipes you may like?

- How easily can you stay on this diet during parties, holidays, time crunches, high-stress periods, and meals with friends?
- How easily can you stick with this diet if the rest of your household is not dieting?

Key facts to know before cutting out carbs

Eating a low-carbohydrate diet for a year can help you lose weight and modestly improve risk factors for heart disease. Unfortunately, it also may increase your risk for cancer depending on your age. So it pays to understand the benefits and risks of cutting out carbs.

Keeps hunger at bay. Low-carb diets restrict carbohydrates like pasta, fruits, and some vegetables, but not protein foods like eggs, cheese, and meat. Protein makes you feel full, so low-carb diets that are high in protein may help you feel less hungry throughout the day.

Some low-carb diets fight hunger by emphasizing foods low on the glycemic index. These include foods like lentils that take longer to digest and won't make your blood sugar skyrocket. To learn more about the glycemic index, see the chapter *Diabetes: outwit a deadly diagnosis*.

Raises cancer risk for some adults. Your body needs protein to function, but a new study suggests eating too much protein could be harmful to adults ages 50 to 65.

Participants in that age range who ate a high- or moderate-protein diet had a much higher risk of dying from cancer than people who ate a low-protein diet. They also were much more likely to die earlier — from any cause — than low-protein dieters. Eating plant-based protein instead of animal protein was less dangerous, and sometimes eliminated the risks.

On the other hand, study participants over age 65 benefited from eating more protein. Compared with a low-protein diet, eating a high-protein diet drastically reduced their odds of dying from any cause within 18 years. Experts warn that more research is needed to determine whether a high-protein diet truly affects your risk of dying early. Check with your doctor for the latest information.

Boosts production of ketones. Drastically reducing carbohydrates can raise your body's production of acidic compounds called ketone bodies. When ketone bodies build up in your bloodstream, that's called ketosis. High levels of ketone bodies may alter your body's acid-alkaline balance enough to endanger your life. Ketosis can be particularly risky for people with heart disease, diabetes, or kidney problems.

Contributes to kidney problems. A high-protein diet may trigger body changes that raise your risk of eventual kidney disease and kidney stones, a recent animal study suggests. If you have kidney disease or diabetes, even a short-term high-protein diet may cause damage from kidney disease to accelerate.

Yields uncertain long-term benefits. Scientists haven't determined whether people on low-carbohydrate, high-protein diets can keep losing weight after one year, or even avoid regaining pounds they've lost. And though one year on a low-carb diet can help improve risk factors for heart disease, no one knows whether those benefits will continue or disappear as time goes on.

Some experts recommend you only use this diet on a short-term basis and under your doctor's supervision. Then switch to a diet that's more nutritionally balanced.

The truth you never hear about fad diets

Just because a diet becomes the latest trend doesn't mean it won't work. But watch out for diets that promise dramatic weight loss with little effort, limit your food choices, or require you to spend a lot of money. Here's what ads for those fad diets won't tell you.

- The pounds may come off quickly at first, but fad diets can't deliver weight loss that lasts, experts say. That's why each one is replaced by another fly-by-night diet that's just as wildly popular.
- Fad diets may keep you from getting enough of certain nutrients such as iron, calcium, zinc, and vitamin B12. If you're deficient in a nutrient long enough, you may develop problems like abnormal heart rhythms, bone loss, kidney stones, or high cholesterol.
- Your body may need more calories than the diet allows, so you may feel unusually tired.
- Fad diets can make you lose weight too quickly, causing symptoms like headaches, constipation, or dizziness. Rapid weight loss can also raise your risk of other dangers, such as problems with dehydration, blood pressure, kidneys, and thyroid.

Don't believe the advertising hype that promises to magically melt away your extra pounds. Make sure any diet you follow provides the nutrition you need to stay healthy while you lose weight.

Avoid dangerous diet-drug combo

Before you try grapefruit at every meal to help slim down, ask your pharmacist if grapefruit can interact dangerously with your prescription medications. Grapefruit may affect cholesterol-lowering statin drugs like atorvastatin (Lipitor); heart medications called calcium channel blockers like nifedipine (Procardia XL, Nifediac, Afeditab, Adalat CC); cyclosporine (Neoral, Sandimmune); anti-anxiety drugs like buspirone (Buspar), and many other prescription drugs.

Watch out for slippery weight-loss scams

That weight-loss product may offer ads showing people in lab coats, an "official" website, and claims like "guaranteed" and "scientific breakthrough." Some scammers even set up fake news sites with logos of familiar news outlets to make their product seem legitimate. To help spot scams that may steal your money or fad diets that may be dangerous, watch for signs like these.

- Claims you'll lose more than 2 pounds a week.
- Blames weight gain on a particular food group, nutrient, or ingredient, and limits food choices.
- Recommends using a single food to promote weight loss.
- Bases claims on little more than "before and after" photos, anecdotal stories, or testimonials.
- Promises quick, easy weight loss through a gimmick that sounds too good to be true — particularly if you won't need to exercise or diet and can eat as much of your favorite "bad" foods as you want.
- Recommends a cream to apply or item to wear to lose weight.
- Requires you to buy special products you can't get at your supermarket, or high-priced seminars, pills, or prepackaged meals.
- Doesn't mention possible risks of the product or diet.
- Guarantees everyone who uses it will lose weight.

5 mind-blowing facts about supplements

Some weight-loss supplements and herbal preparations may come with extra surprises never mentioned in their ads or labels. Here are five startling examples.

The active ingredient may not work. Experts say no scientific studies have shown that the supplement ingredients *Hoodia gordonii* or *Cha de Bugre* help people lose weight. These are advertised as appetite suppressants.

The supplement may contain banned drugs. In 2014, the Food and Drug Administration (FDA) warned against taking several brands of weight-loss supplements because they contained banned medications. The first medication, sibutramine (Meridia), was removed from the market in 2010 because it significantly raises the risk of heart attack and stroke in some people. The second drug, phenolphthalein, is a laxative and suspected cancer-causing drug the FDA has never approved.

It may not be safe to use with your prescriptions. Weight-loss supplement ingredients like bitter orange and diuretics can interact with prescription drugs.

You may face dangerous side effects. Consider these examples.

- Some diet herbal teas or supplements include stimulant laxatives like senna or cascara sagrada. Long-term use of these may lead to dehydration, electrolyte imbalance, kidney failure, and sometimes death.
- Products containing tiratricol, a thyroid hormone, may increase your risk of thyroid problems, heart attack, and stroke.
- Diet supplements that include large amounts of stimulants like caffeine may cause symptoms such as high blood pressure, irregular heart rhythms, nausea, and sleep problems.

Labels may not be correct. Some labels may not list amounts of ingredients or may list an inaccurate amount.

You won't find these problems in every weight-loss supplement, but many are unproven or unsafe. That's why experts recommend you avoid using them and rely on diet and exercise for safer, smarter weight loss.

Diet pills: safe way to shed pounds?

Prescription weight-loss drugs have the benefit of a doctor's supervision, but don't be fooled into thinking they're an easy or safe way to shed unwanted pounds. The Food and Drug Administration (FDA) has approved several new obesity drugs in recent years even though they have questions about side effects. Learn what to expect before you choose one. Ask your doctor these questions.

- Am I a good candidate for a weight-loss drug? Obesity drugs are generally recommended for people with a BMI of 30 or higher. They're also suggested for those with a BMI of 27 or higher who have a serious medical condition, like diabetes or high blood pressure, that could be helped by losing weight.
- Do I still need to diet and exercise? Yes, but these drugs may make cutting calories easier than before. Most obesity drugs suppress your appetite, but one keeps you from absorbing fat. People who overeat due to stress may do better with the fat blocker.
- How long can I take these drugs? Some are approved for long-term use, but others should only be taken for a few months. People often regain weight once they stop using an obesity drug, but making permanent changes to your eating and exercise habits may help keep the weight off.
- What will the drug cost? That depends on whether it's covered by insurance. Ask your insurer if your plan covers the medication and how to qualify for that coverage.

You need a doctor's prescription for these drugs because of possible interactions from your other medications or medical conditions. Your doctor can help you avoid those dangers. Here are a few key facts about each drug to help you narrow your options. Talk to your doctor or pharmacist to learn more.

Drug	Key facts you should know
Fat blockers	
Xenical (orlistat)	You must take a vitamin supplement because you absorb less of the fat-soluble vitamins A, D, E, and K. Eating too much fat may result in diarrhea, leakage of oily stools, and other digestive symptoms. Severe liver injury has been reported in people taking Xenical.
Appetite suppressants	
Adipex-P (phentermine)	May raise blood pressure and heart rate and contribute to insomnia and nervousness. Use is limited to three months because it can be addictive.
Belviq (lorcaserin)	If you haven't lost at least 5 percent of your body weight after 12 weeks, stop taking it because it probably won't work. A few experts have raised concerns about possible heart risks with this drug. Tell your doctor if you take medications for depression, migraines, or erectile dysfunction.
Qsymia (topiramate/ phentermine HCL)	If you haven't lost at least 5 percent of your body weight after 12 weeks on the highest dosage, it probably won't work. A few experts have raised concerns about possible heart risks with this drug. Tell your doctor if you've had a heart attack, stroke, kidney or liver problems, depression or other mood problems, or epilepsy.
Contrave (bupropion/ naltrexone)	Approved by the FDA in 2014 on condition that manufacturer would investigate heart-related risks, possible drug interactions, and appropriate dosage for those with kidney and liver problems. Can raise blood pressure and heart rate so it can't be used by people with uncontrolled high blood pressure.

Beware the risks of nonprescription Alli

Alli is a half-strength version of Xenical (orlistat) you can buy without a prescription. Unfortunately, this means your doctor doesn't pre-check the medicine to help you avoid side effects, drug interactions, and other dangers.

To protect yourself, don't take Alli if you have gallbladder disease, difficulty digesting food, or if you've had an organ transplant. If your doctor says you can't take Xenical, you shouldn't take Alli either. Both drugs have the same active ingredient and carry similar risks.

Before buying or using Alli, complete these safety checks:

- Ask your pharmacist if any prescription drugs you take may interact with Alli.
- Read the information on Xenical in the story *Diet pills: safe way to shed pounds?* It applies to Alli, too.
- Ask your doctor whether you can take Alli safely.

Handy guide to weight-loss surgery

Bariatric weight-loss surgery doesn't remove fat from your body like liposuction does, but it may help shed stubborn pounds after other weight-loss methods fail. Just remember, no operation is risk free. So before talking to your doctor about surgery, learn as much about it as you can. Start with these questions.

Who is eligible for surgery? You may qualify if your body mass index (BMI) is 40 or more, or you're a woman more than 80 pounds overweight or a man more than 100 pounds overweight. You also must have been unable to lose weight using diet, exercise, and medications. You may also qualify if your BMI is at least 35 and you have a serious, obesity-related condition like diabetes, severe arthritis, or high blood pressure.

What are the risks? Your doctor can explain serious risks, but possible complications include hernias, higher risk of vitamin and mineral deficiencies, and leaks or narrowing where the stomach meets your small intestine. You're also at risk for dumping syndrome, a combination of vomiting, reflux, and diarrhea. These problems are more likely if you're over age 45, have a BMI of 50 or higher, or have medical conditions like diabetes.

Will I still need to diet? Weight-loss surgery won't end the need to diet or exercise. Yet studies suggest people who have this surgery are more likely to lose weight and see obesity-related conditions improve during the 10 years after surgery. For example, surgery may reduce your cancer risk, lower blood pressure and cholesterol, and raise your odds of reversing diabetes and sleep apnea. After surgery, you will:

- eat a restricted diet.
- need vitamin and mineral supplements.
- have less tolerance for fat, sugar, and alcohol.
- have to eat more slowly, avoid large meals, and eat smaller amounts to prevent nausea and vomiting.
- have more risk of osteoporosis due to nutrient deficiencies the surgery may cause.

What types of surgery are available? You have a number of procedures to choose from, and your doctor will help you decide which is best for you. These are the three most common.

- Laparoscopic gastric banding. The surgeon attaches a small band around the upper part of your stomach. This creates a small stomach pouch that limits the amount you can eat. The band can be expanded or reduced after surgery, as needed. This surgery is reversible, and nearly 25 percent of people need the band removed later due to problems.
- Vertical banded gastroplasty (gastric partitioning). Using staples and an inflexible band, your surgeon divides the stomach into a small pouch and a larger stomach chamber. Only a little food at a time can pass from the pouch to the stomach chamber.
- Gastric bypass surgery. The surgeon staples the stomach to create a small stomach pouch where food can enter and a larger stomach area that is closed off. Your surgeon also connects your small intestine to the pouch so food can leave your stomach and continue digesting. You'll absorb fewer calories and lose more weight than with gastric banding.

Step 4: Get up and move

Take a stand for health

Have you heard the latest catch phrase? "Sitting is the new smoking."

According to some experts, a sedentary lifestyle — too much sitting and too little exercise — could kill you at about the same rate as smoking. This might be a slight exaggeration, but there's no denying the impact a couch-potato lifestyle has on your health.

Every hour you spend sitting increases the odds you'll develop some kind of condition that will limit your ability to function independently — by a whopping 46 percent.

In other words, the more you simply sit around doing nothing, the more likely it is you'll eventually only be able to do nothing. You'll lose the strength you need to get around the house and perform everyday activities, like preparing food and taking care of yourself.

It makes sense. It's even one of the basic principles you learned in high school science — a body at rest tends to stay at rest. Only now it's more that a body in the recliner tends to stay in the recliner.

Do you know the symptoms of what is sometimes called sitting disease? They include fatigue, weight gain, unsteadiness, weakness, and a lack of flexibility. In addition, without the feel-good hormones your body releases during exercise, called endorphins, you may feel generally lethargic and depressed.

Even more alarming, a lack of exercise whittles away at your good health in ways you may not notice for years — increasing your risk of heart disease, obesity, diabetes, cancer, and even early death.

It doesn't take much to turn this around. Start by getting up. Stand while you clip coupons. Pace when you're on the phone. Move just a little, at first. Learn to listen to your body so you know when to safely ratchet your activity up a level. Know when to push and when to stop.

Find out what fuels your body most efficiently during exercise and what everyday activities give you the most fitness bang for your buck. Most of all, remember, exercise isn't about pain or competition. It's about living.

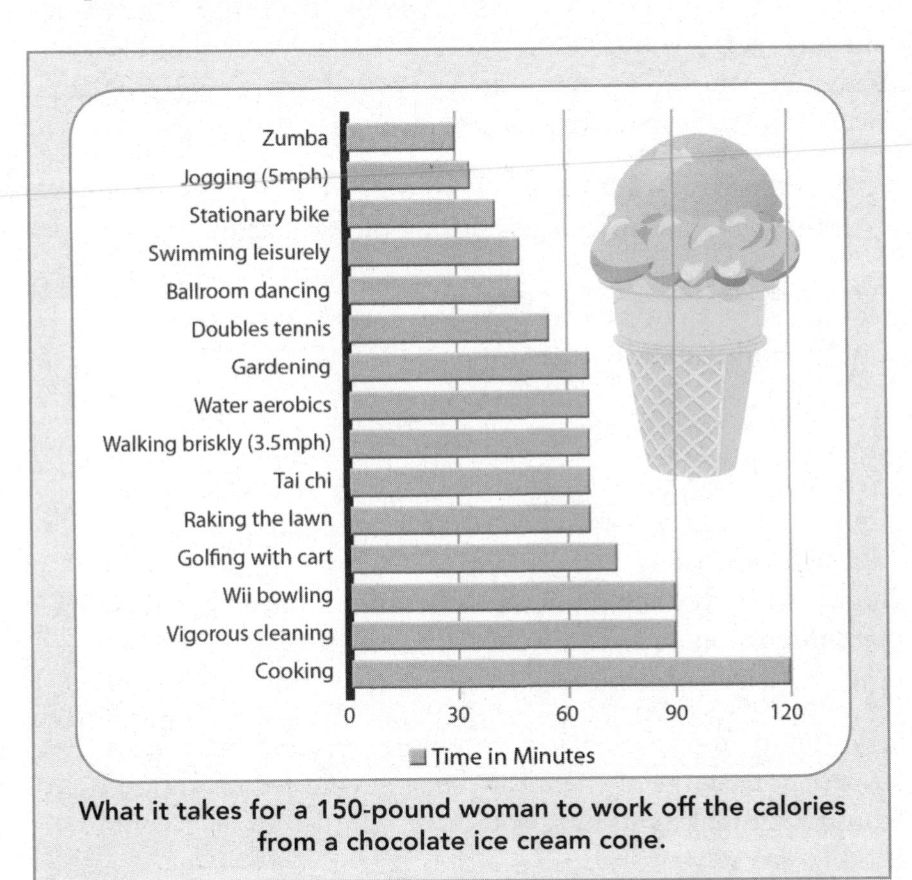

What it takes for a 150-pound woman to work off the calories from a chocolate ice cream cone.

Get ready to get fit

Rediscover the fountain of youth

What does it mean to be physically fit? Don't worry about marathons. Forget Mr. Universe. It's so much simpler than that. It really means you have what it takes to carry out your daily activities. Since that covers a lot of ground, most experts agree overall fitness is made up of these elements:

- cardiorespiratory fitness — your heart and lungs provide the fuel your body needs during physical activity
- muscle strength and endurance
- flexibility and balance
- body composition

When you exercise, your entire body gets involved. Muscles squeeze, lungs expand and contract, and blood pumps furiously through your veins. You know you're working out simply by how your body feels. And yes, sometimes it hurts. But there's a lot more going on than you realize.

During physical activity, extra blood and oxygen course through your brain. You immediately feel more alert and focused and experience a surge of chemicals, such as endorphins and serotonin, that make you feel good.

Your heart beats faster to pump extra blood to your muscles and other tissues. Your lungs swell with oxygen as you breathe harder and faster. Work out often, and you'll increase the efficiency of your heart and lungs, giving you more energy to complete your daily tasks.

Scientists have proven regular exercise helps reduce or even reverse physical losses and aging. In fact, research suggests you can gain back much of the strength, balance, flexibility, and coordination you had when you were much younger — even if you're over 90 years old.

A study of frail 90-year-olds showed they improved their strength, power, and muscle mass, plus had fewer falls, after just 12 weeks of strength and balance training. Maintaining your fitness is a good way to stay healthy and independent into your 90s.

In fact, just 30 minutes of light to moderate physical activity a day is all it takes to add years to your life. That's what British and Swedish researchers found when they reviewed 22 studies comparing physical activity and the risk of early death.

An Australian study found the benefits of exercise even applied to older men through their 80s. Those who got 30 minutes of exercise five days a week were healthier and less likely to die during the 11-year follow-up than men who were sedentary. And a British study found that people in their 70s and 80s who stayed active needed fewer prescriptions and emergency treatment.

Don't worry if you've been a couch potato all your life. The English Longitudinal Study of Aging has shown that people who start exercising late in life also reap significant health benefits. Participants over age 63 who switched to an active lifestyle were less likely to develop chronic disease, depression, physical disability, or memory problems if they stayed active during the eight years they were studied.

Fitness is not just about firm muscles, endless energy, or a trim waistline. It's about giving your body the weapons it needs to fight off both diseases and aging. Every time you exercise to make your body more fit, you may be one step closer to improving your health — or even saving your life. It's like dipping into your very own fountain of youth.

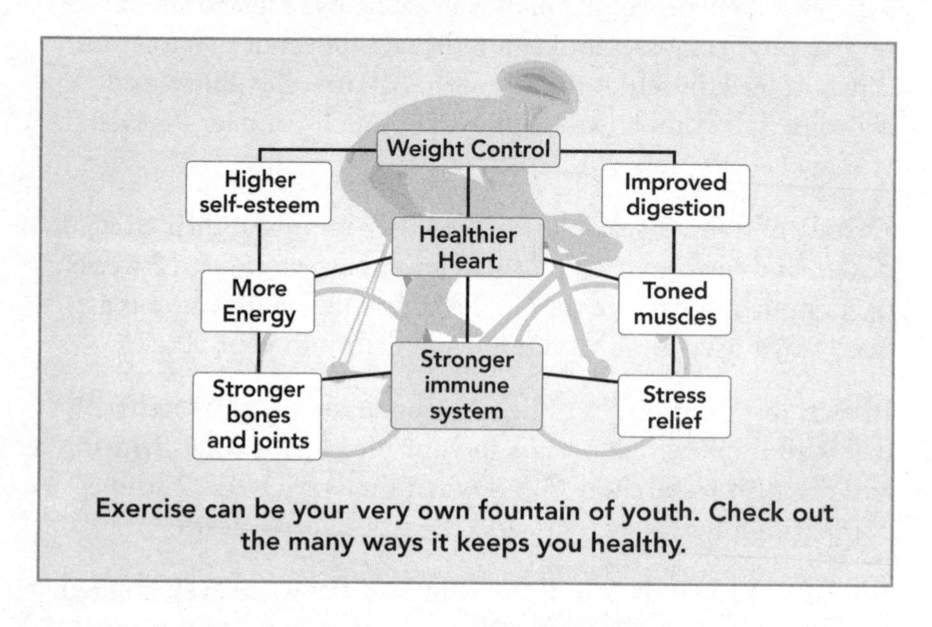

Exercise can be your very own fountain of youth. Check out the many ways it keeps you healthy.

Reap big rewards with a little exercise

What you do today can affect your life decades in the future. A recent German study concluded that if you want to defeat disease, it helps to develop healthy habits at a young age. But it's never too late to start. Physical activity is packed with perks that can make you happier and healthier. Here are a few of its amazing benefits.

Fights fatigue. You may think you don't have the energy to exercise now that you're older, but exercise will actually give you a natural energy boost. Even a 10-minute workout may foil fatigue because it releases chemicals in your brain that improve your mood.

Recharges your metabolism. As you grow older, your metabolism slows down and you burn fewer calories. If you still eat the same number of calories every day — but burn fewer of them — you can't help but gain weight. If only you could find a way to speed that metabolism back up.

Exercise, like strength training, can help. While you're building muscle, you're also revitalizing your metabolism, which can help you lose weight and make you stronger. It's a three-for-one deal that could literally lighten your load.

You'll learn just how easy and beneficial strength training can be when you read No. 1 way to power up your health in the *Stay strong to stop the clock* chapter.

Fires up your immunity. Keep your immune system humming at full power and you're less likely to get sick. Regular, moderate exercise can make sure your immune system stays charged up by stimulating natural killer T cells. They circulate throughout your body fighting invaders like viruses and bacteria. Another plus — your body temperature rises during exercise, which also helps fight off germs.

Tunes up your digestive system. If you're plagued by poor digestion, the answer may be at your feet. A daily brisk walk — or any other moderate exercise — can ease constipation enough that you can throw away those pills and powders. This "natural laxative" can help your digestive system work smoothly — without any of the unpleasant side effects that come from harsh laxatives.

Powers up your heart. Heart attack, stroke, high cholesterol, and high blood pressure are all serious heart-related conditions. Yet physical activity can lower your risk for all of them.

Exercise has been proven to cut triglycerides and total cholesterol and keep resting blood pressure rates lower for hours after an exercise session ends. And a recent study says exercise may work even better than drugs when it comes to fighting heart attack and stroke. Researchers found it especially effective at fending off a second attack in stroke and heart attack survivors.

How to add fitness to your life — and love it

Anyone can exercise. Whether you're 8 or 80, you can find an activity that gets you moving and makes you feel good. With just a few preparations, you'll be ready to work out with the best of them — at your own pace.

Get motivated. Before you jump into a fitness program, figure out what's motivating you. Your goal may be to lose weight and look better, but you're more apt to succeed if you focus on changing your lifestyle and improving your health.

Make your first experience a positive one to help motivate you to keep it up. Researchers found that students with a positive memory of exercise were more likely to continue working out than those who held a negative memory or no memory at all. If you need more of a push, try some of these ideas:

- Choose activities you enjoy that fit easily into your daily schedule.
- Try new sports, games, or exercises from time to time so you won't get bored.
- Listen to recorded books or music while you work out. Check your local library for CDs you might enjoy.
- Find an exercise buddy — or even a group or club. Having someone to exercise with can encourage you and keep you from giving up.

Come up with a plan. Think about where you want to work out. You can exercise at home, but if you like organized exercise, try a gym or health club. It's best to learn from a trainer or class instructor to be sure you know how to do the exercise correctly. You'll get better results and suffer fewer injuries.

Decide on a regular exercise time, and block it off on your calendar. Be sure to include time for warming up and cooling down. Don't forget to have a back-up plan. For example, keep an exercise DVD or video handy for those days when weather, travel, or even house guests prevent your usual outdoor exercise or trip to the gym.

Seek expert advice. Your doctor can be your greatest champion in your quest for fitness. In fact, before you begin any exercise, talk with him about the best activities for you. Ask if any of your health conditions or medications could affect your exercise plans and if you should avoid specific activities.

Make exercise part of your day. Routine tasks such as cleaning the house, gardening, and washing the car can increase your fitness level at home. But for more of a challenge, add aerobic activities like walking, jogging, biking, swimming, and tennis. Even sex and dancing count as healthy exercise. Both burn calories and give your muscles a workout, plus they're great ways to involve your spouse.

Research shows that aerobic exercise helps protect your brain from shrinking, so these seven activities are super ways to slow or even reverse the aging process. To learn more about the positive ways exercise affects your brain, see *Beat the blues and think sharper, too* in the *Cardio: surprising moves to change your life* chapter.

Ramp up your efforts. Older adults should aim for two and a half hours of moderate physical activity or an hour and 15 minutes of vigorous exercise every week. Research shows that exercising a minimum of three days a week will produce health benefits.

If you haven't been active in the past, work your way up so you eventually replace some moderate activities with tougher workouts. The easiest way is to exercise either longer or more often. If you normally walk or bike 30 minutes three times a week, push yourself to 50 to 60 minutes. Or extend your workout to five days a week.

Setting a higher goal may be just the challenge you need to keep going until you reach a point where exercise becomes second nature. Then you'll do it because you love it.

Antioxidants can sabotage your workout

You take supplements because you think they'll give you an edge in your quest for fitness. After all, antioxidants attack those nasty free radicals that cause aging and disease, so the more, the better, right?

Not so fast. Recent studies have cautioned that antioxidants may work against you during exercise because your body needs oxidative stress caused by free radicals to perform.

A study of Norwegian runners and cyclists who trained intensely for 11 weeks found that those who took large doses of vitamins C and E had significantly lower levels of energy markers than those taking a placebo. Until scientists learn more, you may want to ditch the supplements and rely on natural foods for your vitamins.

And a Danish study of older men discovered that the natural compound resveratrol found in red grapes and wine blocks many of exercise's heart-protective benefits. These include lowering blood pressure and cholesterol.

Top eating tips for an active lifestyle

There's no denying you are what you eat. And no matter how old you are, good nutrition is important. In fact, for healthy aging, eating right goes hand in hand with exercise.

Food fuels your body, so proper nutrition is essential to your fitness program. You need nutrients to build muscles and strengthen bones, as well as stay active all day long.

Just remember, if you're doing light to moderate workouts, you don't need extra calories. Experts say many people overestimate how many calories they've burned and treat themselves to too many rich snacks.

Energize with carbohydrates. Your body runs on glucose, which comes from carbohydrates. Glucose is stored in your muscles as glycogen, so giving your body a good supply of carbs is essential for energy. Focus on eating high-quality carbohydrates like whole-grain breads, pasta, cereal, fruits, and vegetables.

Power up with protein. You need protein to build and repair muscle. Your body also relies on protein for energy if you don't get enough carbohydrates. Lean beef, pork, or chicken are good meat choices, but you can also get protein from dairy as well as beans and other legumes.

Focus on nutrient-packed foods. Look for foods that give you the most nutritional bang for your buck, filled with the vitamins and minerals you need. Any deficiencies can affect your performance no matter what activities you're involved in.

If you find you're always tired, for example, you may be low in vitamin B-12. This powerhouse vitamin is involved in many of your body's key functions. It's easy to get by eating fish, red meat, milk, yogurt, and eggs.

Drink plenty of water. It's important to stay hydrated, but skip the high-priced sports drinks unless you're working out intensely for more than an hour. Two hours before a workout, drink about two cups of water, then continue to sip during and after your exercise. Keep a water bottle with you, and use it frequently throughout the day.

Know what and when to eat. Experts usually recommend eating a carbohydrate-rich meal two to four hours before exercising. But a recent study suggests eating a high-protein meal before exercising moderately for 30 minutes will help you burn calories more effectively.

To restore your glycogen supply and repair muscles after your workout, eat a snack with carbohydrates and protein, preferably within 30 minutes. Try a glass of fat-free chocolate milk or a turkey sandwich.

Simple ways to guarantee success

Finding out how fit you are — or even how fit you aren't — helps you tailor a fitness plan to your needs. After all, no adult is typical. So don't worry if you're not a tough-as-nails athlete. Simply become more active, and you'll start feeling the benefits and seeing the results. Here are some ways to make sure you succeed.

Evaluate your fitness level. Grab a notebook, and write down how much time you spend exercising or being physically active each day. Monitor yourself for a week, and include activities like housework, yardwork, or walking around a shopping mall.

To get a rough measure of your aerobic, strength, and flexibility fitness, try these fitness tests recommended by the Mayo Clinic. Go to *www.mayoclinic.org*, and search on "measuring fitness." Check with your doctor before you begin. He may want you to take a stress test to make sure your heart is strong enough for vigorous exercise.

Set goals to improve. Does your log tell you you're less active than you thought? Are you on the low end of the aerobic fitness scale? Now is the time to set goals and focus on where you want to be in six months or a year.

Pick realistic goals that are important to you for the best chance of success. For example, in six months you will lower your blood pressure five points, lose 20 pounds, or walk two miles with your dog.

Track your efforts. Now comes the fun part, especially if you like gadgets. To monitor your fitness, you can use something as simple as a pedometer to count your steps or as complex as a wristband sensor that collects and analyzes your personal data.

These state-of-the-art devices can tell you everything from how many calories you've burned to how well you've slept, and measure your heart rate, sweat, and body temperature to boot. Have a smartphone or tablet? You can choose from a multitude of free apps that collect this information and give you instant feedback for on-the-spot motivation. Some of the more popular apps and fitness gadgets include MyFitnessPal, LoseIt, RunKeeper, Argus, Fitbit, and Jawbone UP.

If technological toys leave your head spinning, just remember this. The best device is one you're willing to wear, helps you understand your activity level, and motivates you to be more active throughout the day. Other features may be helpful, but they're not necessarily better. Read user reviews in magazines like *PC World* or *PC Magazine*, or talk to someone at your local tech store, to help you choose a device that's right for you.

To make it even simpler, track your fitness the old-fashioned way. Each week, write down your exercise goals at the top of a notebook page, for example, three hours of aerobic activity. Make a chart listing the days of the week, and for each day, list what exercise you did, how vigorous the effort, and how long your session lasted. At the end of the week, you can total your hours and see if you've met your goal. Doesn't get any easier than that.

4 ways to tell if it's a good workout

Strive for 150 minutes of moderate exercise or 75 minutes of vigorous exercise every week, or a combination of the two. That's what experts recommend, but how do you know if you're getting it right?

The best way to tell if you're getting the most from your workout is to figure out how much energy you're burning while you exercise. These techniques can help.

Know your MET activity score. Scientists use something called a metabolic equivalent (MET) to classify the intensity of activities. The baseline is 1 MET, which is how much energy you use while sitting quietly.

Moderate-intensity activities are defined as 3.0 to 5.9 METs, which means you exert about three to six times more energy than you do at rest. Walking 3 mph, playing doubles tennis, or ballroom dancing would put you in this category.

Vigorous activities are 6.0 METs and above. Running a 10-minute mile is a 10 MET activity classified as vigorous. Others include bicycling more than 10 mph, singles tennis, and step aerobics.

To get the health benefits your body needs, experts recommend you get 500 to 1,000 MET minutes per week. To figure that out, simply multiply the MET activity number times the number of minutes you exercise. For example, if you do a 10 MET activity for 50 minutes, you'll achieve 500 MET minutes and meet your minimum weekly goal. You can find MET activity scores on various websites.

Measure your heart rate. Many people gauge their exercise intensity through target heart rate, a technique that tells you how fast your heart should beat during exercise. According to the American Heart Association, your target heart rate range should fall between 50 percent and 85 percent of your maximum heart rate. Look for details on how to figure out your target heart rate in the *Cardio: surprising moves to change your life* chapter.

Tune in to your body. If you take medication or have a condition that changes your heart rate, you're better off listening to your body to determine how hard you're working. The Borg Rating of Perceived Exertion Scale can help you do that.

The scale features numbered levels that describe how hard you're exercising based on how you feel. For endurance activities, you should work your way up to level 13, which is "somewhat hard." For strength training, you would aim for level 17, or "very hard." As you become more fit, you'll find you need more challenging activities to reach those same levels.

Rely on the talk test. Tired of all those numbers? The easiest way to figure out if you're exercising too hard is by talking with a friend while you work out. If you can hold a conversation, you're doing moderate exercise. Can barely talk? Consider it a vigorous activity. Other ways to tell you're working hard — you'll sweat a lot and your muscles may feel rubbery.

NEAT way to rev up your metabolism

You can burn up to 1,000 calories a day without the gym or a tough workout — just be moving continuously throughout the day.

Nonexercise activity thermogenesis (NEAT) is a fancy way of describing all the things you do every day that aren't considered exercise — like raking leaves, playing the piano, typing, climbing stairs, and doing dishes. NEAT moves like these don't burn a lot of calories on their own, but the numbers add up over the course of a day.

Fidgeting counts as a NEAT activity, but it's not enough to burn many calories. Instead, make an effort to get up and move whenever you can. Pace while talking on the phone, march in place while watching TV, or walk the sidelines of your grandson's soccer game instead of sitting in the bleachers.

Easy does it: no-work workouts

The safest, cheapest exercise you'll love to do anywhere, anytime

Walking doesn't require any special talent or training — you just do it without thinking. Yet if you put a little extra time and effort into it each day, you get amazing results. You lose weight, have more energy, lower your blood pressure and cholesterol, think more clearly, have less anxiety, and sleep a whole lot better. And that's just the beginning.

Benefits like these have turned walking into one of the most popular fitness activities ever. People tend to give up on most exercise programs after the first big push, but walkers are more like the Energizer Bunny — they keep on going. That's because they discover it is a steady, sure way to health and fitness. Research shows that walking is a simple method you can use to reduce or even eliminate your everyday aches and pains. Walkers don't stop when they get older, either. More men over age 65 are regular walkers than in any other age group. For many people, a daily walk has become their ticket to a longer, healthier, more enjoyable life.

Want more reasons to walk? Try these five and see if they don't persuade you to put on your walking shoes right now.

- You can walk just about any time you're in the mood. You don't have to make a reservation, change clothes, or wait for others to join you.

- You can afford it. There are no clubs to join or expensive equipment to buy. All you really need are comfortable clothes and supportive shoes.
- You can adjust your walking schedule around your other activities. If you need a break or have a few spare minutes, take a walk.
- You can do it anywhere — in your own neighborhood or local park, while you're shopping, even when you're out of town. If the weather is bad and you don't want to dress for it, walk indoors. The local mall is an ideal place if you don't have a treadmill.
- You are less likely to get hurt than with other activities. Walking is low impact, so you don't have the stress on your joints that leads to blown-out knees, sprained ankles, and bad backs. Other health risks are almost zero, because it's less strenuous than most activities.

When you start walking for fitness, walk for about 10 minutes a day, a few days a week. Then go for 15 minutes, and eventually work up to longer walks on more days. Once you're getting out regularly, increase your pace to a brisk walk. Aim for a moderately intense pace of about 15 to 16 minutes per mile for the most health benefits. Good technique matters, too. When you walk:

- keep your chin up, your shoulders back, and your belly flat.
- take long, easy strides. Land on your heel, roll forward to the ball of your foot, and push off from your toes.
- breathe deeply and let your arms swing naturally.
- lean forward a little when going fast or up and down hills.

For help with balance or for a more strenuous workout, try using Nordic walking poles. These popular devices can improve your posture and endurance, plus help you burn more calories.

Look for more tips on getting a good aerobic workout in the chapter *Cardio: surprising moves to change your life.*

Improve your mood on the trail

Want to get more from your outdoor walks? Try taking a hike. Head into the woods or out to the country, and walk the trails instead of the sidewalks. Do it with friends, and you'll boost the benefits. A recent study found that group nature walks help relieve stress, lessen depression, and make you feel better all around.

"Walking is an inexpensive, low-risk, and accessible form of exercise. And it turns out that, combined with nature and group settings, it may be a very powerful, underutilized stress buster," says researcher Sara Warber, associate professor of family medicine at the University of Michigan Medical School.

Join an outdoor walking or hiking group, or gather some friends and create one of your own. It's a simple way to feel better mentally and emotionally.

Strong, stretchy muscles in 30 seconds

Stretching is essential for fitness. It maximizes the benefits of walking, strength training, golf, or whatever other activities you enjoy. It's also worth doing for its own sake. The more flexible you are, the easier and more pleasant your everyday activities will be.

Your body tends to lose flexibility as you age, but stretching can slow and even reverse this process. Include it in your exercise regimen, and you'll quickly see a difference. You may become flexible enough to sit on the floor and play with your grandkids. Or you may be able to reach for groceries high on the supermarket shelf without any help. Here are just a few things stretching can do for you.

- Return your full range of motion. That may lead to balance and coordination you haven't had for decades, which could reduce your danger of slipping or falling. Flexible, fit muscles also mean better posture and fewer everyday aches and pains.
- Increase blood flow. More nutrients will reach your muscles, while waste products will get flushed away.
- Reduce your risk for injury. Or, for already injured muscles, stretching could shorten your healing time.
- Relieve painful knots. Stretching is like giving yourself a massage. It helps loosen those knots left behind by the daily grind.

That said, stretching before you exercise won't help your performance and may even be harmful. It's best to stretch after your aerobic or strengthening workout when your muscles are warm. If you do a separate stretching session, warm up beforehand with some light walking or arm pumping.

Stretching should not be difficult or painful. When you stretch, your muscle should only feel slightly uncomfortable. Don't push beyond that. The more you stretch, the easier it will become. To gain the most flexibility, perform your stretching routine three to five days a week. Follow these tips for a safe workout.

- Ease into the stretch and hold it for 10 to 30 seconds. Never bounce or jerk.
- Don't hold your breath. Make sure you breathe naturally throughout the stretch.
- Avoid "locking" your joints when you straighten them.
- Repeat the stretch three times for each muscle, resting between repetitions.

Touch your toes for a healthier heart

Has it been years since you've touched your toes from a sitting position? If so, you may have more to worry about than stiff muscles — you may have stiff blood vessels, too. And that raises your risk for a fatal stroke or heart attack.

By their mid-40s, most people find themselves stretching 3 to 5 inches less in the "sit-and-reach" test because they lose elasticity in their tendons, ligaments, and muscles. And now, researchers have shown a link between poor flexibility and heart disease.

What's the connection? One theory is that the collagen and elastin that make your muscles flexible do the same for your artery walls. By regularly stretching your body and keeping your muscles limber, you may help slow the natural stiffening your arteries undergo as you age.

Forget pills and shots — this works better

Yoga uses a series of gentle fixed poses and stretches to loosen your limbs and calm your mind. It improves your balance and flexibility and aids breathing, so you can practice it no matter what your age, weight, or fitness level.

Enthusiasts agree it is the perfect anti-stress exercise. No running, no sweating, and no heavy weights. Yet yoga is scientifically proven to relieve tension, ease pain, lower blood pressure, boost immunity, and even curb overeating.

Do you suffer from lower back pain? Forget pills and shots. In one study, this twice-a-week remedy eased chronic low back pain better than a doctor's care. And this nonmedical therapy is so effective at reducing blood pressure that many doctors now prescribe it to their patients.

Exciting new research has also shown that doing a basic yoga pose called the side plank on your weaker side can improve scoliosis, a potentially serious spinal condition.

One study reported that doing the side plank for 1.5 minutes a day, six days a week, for two months reduced the curvature in people's spines an average of 32 percent.

The best way to learn how to do yoga poses correctly is through a class with a qualified instructor. A good yoga instructor will help you modify the poses based on your abilities or limitations. Keep these points in mind as you begin.

- You need very little gear for yoga — just comfortable, loose clothing and a mat to protect your back.
- Do the breathing techniques correctly for a successful workout. Follow the breathing instructions for each exercise exactly, and always breathe through your nose.
- Start with some basic moves and concentrate on perfecting them before you move on to harder poses.
- Never bounce, jerk, or push a stretch to the point of pain.
- Tell your yoga teacher if you have osteoporosis, so she can adjust your poses to help you avoid harming fragile bones.
- Get your doctor's OK before beginning yoga if you have high blood pressure, heart disease, or have had a stroke or recent surgery.

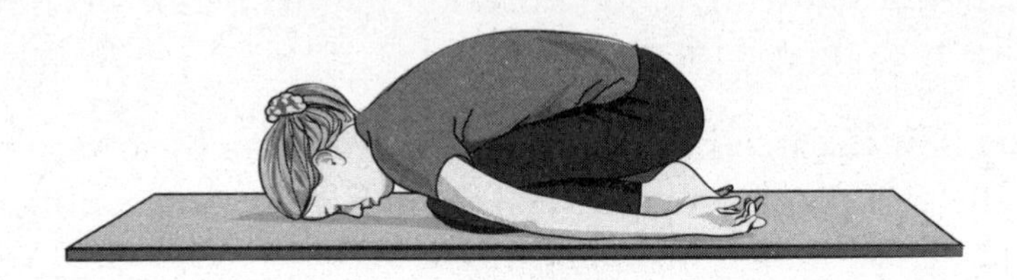

Start your day with the child's pose. You'll stretch all your muscles with this one, simple move and feel great.

- Assume a kneeling position with the tops of your feet against your mat.
- Lower your buttocks until they rest on your heels. If you have difficulty with this position, place a folded blanket between your calves and your buttocks.
- Bend forward and drop your chest onto your thighs. Relax your shoulders and rest your forehead gently on the mat or a pillow.
- Drape your arms loosely at your sides, palms up. Relax and breathe deeply.
- Hold for a minute or two, then return slowly to a sitting position.

Cardio: surprising moves to change your life

Get moving to live longer, feel younger

The beauty of regular aerobic exercise is that you can reap big rewards with relatively little time and effort. All forms of this type of exercise concentrate on fitness and endurance more than strength. And if you stick to low-impact activities without a lot of jarring and strain on your joints, you'll have less wear and tear on your body.

By definition, aerobic exercise uses the oxygen you breathe to produce energy and allow you to work out for a long period of time. Some aerobic activities are jogging, dancing, bicycling, skating, swimming, and even shoveling and mowing.

Walking, of course, is the quickest and easiest way to start an aerobic program, but if you're looking for greater variety or a bigger challenge, there are plenty of other aerobic exercises you can do — and have fun at the same time. Some, like bicycling, involve pushing yourself harder and farther. Others, like water and step aerobics, might mean enrolling in a class.

But it doesn't have to be difficult. Aerobic exercise can be child's play — literally. Play with your kids or grandkids, and you'll blend the fun of a second childhood with healthy exercise. Tag, hide and seek, and kickball are a few old favorites to try, even if you have to adjust the rules a bit for slower, safer play. Any aerobic activity, if done regularly, will improve your overall fitness.

Pumps up your heart and lungs. Aerobic exercise raises your heart rate and keeps it up — at around 70 to 85 percent of your heart rate maximum. (See *The right way to max out your workout* later in this chapter.) This increases the amount of oxygen your body delivers to your muscles. The more oxygen they have, the longer they can work without getting tired. Aerobic exercise strengthens your heart and increases your lungs' ability to gather oxygen, making the whole system more efficient.

Burns away fat. Aerobic exercise is great for weight loss, too. It speeds up your metabolism, which stimulates the fat-burning process. Regular aerobic exercise — two to three times a week — helps you lose fat and gain lean, toned muscle. Your metabolism continues at a faster pace even after you've stopped exercising, so the better you condition your aerobic system, the more fat you burn up.

Ready to start reaping these wonderful benefits? These tips will help guarantee your success.

- Start low and go slow. Choose activities that are appropriate for your current fitness level and health goals. Increase your activity gradually over time.
- Use the right gear for your activity. Buy a good pair of walking or running shoes, get a bicycle helmet, or invest in safety gear for activities like rollerblading or soccer.
- Learn the proper technique. Understand what is involved in your activity, and get help with the proper form if you need it. That will help you perform it correctly and minimize your chances of getting hurt.
- Listen to your body. If you're in pain, stop and rest. It's a sign that something may be wrong.

Run away from vision loss

Your aging eyes can suffer from a number of serious conditions, but an easy exercise like walking can help protect them. Research shows that regular aerobic exercise reduces your risk of developing cataracts, macular degeneration, and glaucoma.

If you can step it up, you'll reap even more protection. In recent studies, men who ran more than 5.7 miles a day slashed their cataract risk by more than one-third compared to men who ran less than 1.4 miles daily.

And for every 0.6 miles people ran every day, their chances of developing age-related macular degeneration dropped 10 percent.

Beat the blues and think sharper, too

Would you believe something as simple as searching for items in an unfamiliar store can sharpen your memory and problem-solving skills? The act of walking and thinking at the same time benefits you more than mental exercise alone.

Aerobic exercise floods your brain cells with oxygen and nutrients. That may be why physical activity can speed your thinking and help you process information faster. It also helps keep your blood vessels from hardening, including those in your brain. Experts think that may be a key reason some people stay mentally sharp as they age.

Working on puzzles and games is a great way to stay mentally fit. But the real secret to boosting your brain is working out the rest of your body, too. Here are some benefits exercise provides.

Fends off dementia. Although most people's brains shrink somewhat as they age, those who have a genetic marker for Alzheimer's disease tend to lose even more volume in the hippocampus, the region of the brain dealing with memory and learning. But moderate exercise seems to have a protective effect.

"We found that physical activity has the potential to preserve the volume of the hippocampus in those with increased risk for Alzheimer's disease," says Dr. J. Carson Smith, a researcher at the University of Maryland School of Public Health. "That means we can possibly delay cognitive decline and the onset of dementia symptoms in these individuals."

Other studies also tout the protective effects of exercise. Dutch scientists found that regular aerobic exercise boosted the size of the hippocampus in women with mild memory problems. And research out of Finland showed that people who exercised twice a week had a lower risk of dementia than those who were less active, even if they started after middle age.

Battles the blues. Whether you occasionally feel down or suffer from more serious depression, exercise can help. When you work out, your body releases endorphins that help you feel good and lowers your level of the stress hormone cortisol.

But it's more than just a feel-good-for-the-moment remedy. Research shows that sports and physical activity actually create changes in the brain similar to mood-altering drugs.

What's more, a Swedish study on mice discovered that exercise raises levels of a muscle enzyme that helps protect the brain against depression. It does this by attacking a particular stress protein and breaking it up before it passes into the brain, where it can affect your mood.

Changes your attitude. Good mental health is having a mindset that expects — and fights for — good health. Regular physical activity can give you the confidence to develop that mindset as well as improve your overall attitude. A recent study found that people who exercise regularly tend to be more positive and more willing to participate in healthy habits following a diagnosis of heart disease. That makes them more likely to live longer than people with heart disease who don't exercise.

CAUTION

New health woes for couch potatoes

It's easy to find excuses not to exercise even though you know it helps every part of your body, including your brain. Unfortunately, a life of laziness changes your brain, too — but not in a good way. And it may have consequences for your heart as well.

A recent animal study showed that a sedentary lifestyle changed the shape of neurons in the brain, making them more sensitive to stimuli. This sensitivity can cause problems with the sympathetic nervous system, which regulates your fight-or-flight response. That, in turn, affects your blood vessels, putting you at risk for high blood pressure and heart disease.

Do yourself a favor, get up off the couch, and start moving. If you sit all day at work, take a break every 10 to 20 minutes, walk around, or do a few jumping jacks. Your brain, and your heart, will thank you.

The right way to max out your workout

Target heart rate is a good way to judge how hard you're working during aerobic exercise. It tells you how fast the average person should make their heart beat to get the best workout.

Several formulas can help you estimate your maximum heart rate, but the simplest one is to subtract your age from 220. From there you can determine your target heart rate for different fitness goals.

For aerobic fitness, experts recommend you exercise at 70 to 85 percent of your maximum heart rate. The following table gives you a general idea where your heart rate should be to achieve that range.

Beats per minute

Age	Target zone	Average max heart rate
40	126 – 153	180
50	119 – 145	170
60	112 – 136	160
70	105 – 128	150
80	98 – 119	140

Keep in mind that you should work up to your target heart rate gradually. One way to make sure you're not progressing too fast is to measure your heart rate when you first start an aerobic activity. For example, if you usually walk a mile, walk it at your normal pace. Take your pulse when you finish, and record your heartbeats per minute.

Each time you walk, try to work harder so your pulse rate gets faster over time. Eventually, you can aim to get your heart rate up to the target 70-to-85-percent range.

For best results, maintain your target heart rate for at least 20 minutes. But don't worry — you don't have to work that hard every time to stay in shape.

Caution — if you have a medical condition or take medicine that changes your heart rate, this might not be the best way to determine your target heart rate. Ask your doctor for advice.

Step up to a healthier you

Step aerobics is an ideal workout because you get the cardiovascular benefits of running but the lower joint stress of walking. It uses the large muscles in your legs and is rhythmic and repetitive, all essentials of aerobic exercise. There's also an element of strength training involved. By raising and lowering the weight of your body, you're building muscles, too.

The simplest way to get started on step aerobics is to go up and down your stairs at home. Another way is to use the bottom stair as a platform. Just step up onto it and back down.

If you want something a little more structured, try a step aerobics class or buy a video to use at home. You'll learn how to properly step onto and off of a low bench or platform. An instructor demonstrates the movements to music and keeps the routine going.

Once you get your footwork down, you can boost the intensity of your workout by adding arm movements. Just don't work your arms above shoulder level for any length of time since this can hurt your shoulders. Rather, change frequently from low- to mid- to high-range movements.

Here are some tips for successful stepping:

- Use good posture — head and chest up, abdominal muscles lightly contracted, and buttocks tucked under your hips.
- Watch the platform when stepping up to make sure you get your entire foot on it. Letting your heel hang over the edge invites Achilles tendon problems.

- Step softly and quietly to avoid stress on your ankles and knees.
- Stay close to the platform when stepping down, and let your heel touch the floor to help absorb the impact.

Small change in training burns more fat

Imagine the opposite of aerobic exercise, and you've got anaerobic exercise. It describes a short burst of vigorous activity — like sprinting, jumping, or lifting weights. Sports like baseball, basketball, and racquetball are also anaerobic activities.

This type of exercise is so demanding, it pushes your heart rate above 85 percent of the maximum level. When this happens, your muscles need more energy than your oxygen supply creates through burning fat. So instead of using oxygen, your body burns stored carbohydrates and protein calories.

Doing some high-intensity intervals in the middle of your run or walk is a good way to add anaerobic exercise to your workout. You'll benefit by burning more calories at rest, developing a leaner body, and increasing your level of fitness. One study showed it even improves blood sugar control in people with type 2 diabetes.

Splash your way to ultimate fitness

Water aerobics can work wonders. Its buoyancy reduces the stress on your weight-bearing joints by as much as 90 percent — cutting down on muscle soreness and injury. Yet water provides the resistance needed to develop a strong heart and lungs.

Plus, new research says that immersing your body in water above your heart increases blood flow to your brain, which may help improve your thinking skills.

General water aerobics classes spend about 10 minutes stretching and then do routines with dumbbells, belts, and ankle straps that serve as both flotation and resistance devices. They also walk and run in the water and do exercises while suspended in the water.

If you want a more solitary water exercise and don't need the structure of a class, just go swimming. When you swim laps, you work almost every muscle in your body.

Whether you decide to take a class or just swim for fitness, you'll want the right equipment, facility, and instruction.

- Purchase a swimsuit that fits well and doesn't restrict your movements.
- A swim cap will protect your hair from sun and chemicals and keep it out of your eyes.
- For swimming laps, a pair of goggles helps keep water and chemicals out of your eyes and improves your underwater vision.
- When choosing a place to swim, look around the facility to see if it's clean and well maintained. Is the staff friendly, helpful, and knowledgeable?
- Talk to the instructor before you sign up for a class. Ask if she can recommend a specific class to help you reach your goals.

You can find water aerobics classes through local recreation departments, the YMCA or YWCA, or fitness clubs and gyms. Many country club and neighborhood pools also offer classes.

Stay strong to stop the clock

No. 1 way to power up your health

You don't have to be Charles Atlas to power up with strength training. This kind of exercise is a key to fitness for everyone — especially seniors.

Lifting weights can help you stay active, build strong bones, and keep your joints limber and pain-free. And stronger muscles and bones could help you preserve your mobility and independence.

Recent research found that 90-year-olds who strength trained for three months were able to walk faster and get out of their chairs more easily, had better balance and fewer falls, and showed more strength in their legs.

Revitalize muscles and bones. When you follow a regular lifting program, you'll start seeing muscles you haven't seen since you were 30 years old. Strength training carves muscles until they become lean and well-defined. It gets results by "stressing" your muscles, which causes tiny microscopic tears in the muscle fibers. As your body repairs them, it adds extra protein to make the muscle stronger.

Lifting weights can also build up your bones. When muscles flex during strength training, the bones around them respond like plants to sunlight — they grow. Stronger muscles also take the stress off your joints and make them more stable. One study found that weight training helped relieve the pain of knee arthritis.

Burn up calories. Unlike fat, muscles do more than take up space. They're constantly eating up calories — three times as many as fat. They keep churning even when you're not exercising. The more you strength train, the more muscles you'll build, which will help your body burn fat faster. So add some muscle and watch the fat melt away.

Cut risk of diabetes. Middle-age and older women who "pump iron" may help cut their risk of developing type 2 diabetes, researchers say. Data from two Nurses Health studies following nearly 100,000 women showed that weightlifting women were less likely to develop diabetes than those who did no weight-bearing exercise. This was true even if they did no aerobic exercise.

Save your memory. Best of all, lifting weights may help improve and protect your thinking and memory well into your senior years. One study found that elderly women who took strength training classes twice weekly for a year boosted their mental function significantly. A study of memory-impaired women reported similar results after only six months. And young, healthy adults who did an intense 20-minute weight workout remembered 10 percent more than those not lifting weights when tested two days later.

To reap the benefits of strength training, you need to exercise all your major muscle groups, including your legs, hips, back, chest, stomach, shoulders, and arms. You can use stretchy resistance bands or even common items like bags of rice, soup cans, or bottled water if you don't have traditional weights. Body-weight exercises like pushups and sit-ups count as well.

Repeat each exercise 8 to15 times, and do your workout at least two days a week. Check with your doctor before starting.

- Use small weights to start out, gradually increasing as you progress. You need to challenge your muscles but don't want to injure yourself.
- Take three seconds to lift the weight, hold for one second, then lower for a count of three.

- Use slow, steady movements. Don't jerk or thrust weights into position, and don't let them drop.
- Breathe normally. Holding your breath can raise your blood pressure.
- Avoid "locking" your elbows or knees in an overly straightened position.
- Don't cross your legs or bend your hips more than 90 degrees if you've had a hip replacement.

Save yourself from a life-altering injury

How steady are you when you stand with your feet together or turn in a circle? Can you quickly get up from a chair without using your arms?

If your balance is a bit wobbly, you have a higher risk of falling. In fact, people age 65 and older have a one-in-three chance of falling during the year.

Learning how to prevent falls can save you from a serious injury, which can affect your independence. Practicing balance exercises can help. But if you do start to fall, here are four things to do.

- Take a quick step or two to catch your balance.
- Grab onto someone or something to help break your fall.
- Roll out of the fall as you drop.
- Fall forward or backward instead of falling on your hip. Breaking a hip can lead to extended hospitalization and even death.

Flatten a bulging belly in 10 workouts

You can stretch and lengthen your muscles with a slow, graceful, and best of all, low-impact Pilates workout. Pilates is so effective it will even help flatten your bulging belly and strengthen your back, while improving your posture and balance.

Traditional Pilates is a combination of mat work and machine-aided exercises, but you can do either one alone. The mat work is easy to learn and can be practiced anywhere. All you need is a good exercise mat and comfortable clothing. Socks or bare feet work best.

Pilates moves focus on developing your core, which includes the deep abdominal muscles and the muscles closest to your spine. But the workout is vigorous enough to qualify as a strength-training program. You will see speedy results — many people notice a difference after just 10 to 20 sessions.

For the most tummy-flattening benefit, combine your Pilates exercises with aerobic workouts. Pilates strengthens and tones your abdominal muscles, while calorie-burning cardio lowers your overall body fat.

Whether you participate in a Pilates class or video, keep these points in mind.

- Tuck in your tummy while doing Pilates moves. Draw the muscles in your abdomen toward your spine, sort of like pulling in to zip up tight pants. If you tighten your lower back and buttocks muscles at the same time, it's called "engaging your powerhouse."
- When you're told to lift your head off the mat, keep a bit of space between your chin and chest, and always look straight ahead. If this is difficult, you can leave your head down, or prop it on a towel or cushion.

- Don't hold your breath during any exercise. Keep breathing deeply the entire time — in through your nose and out through your mouth.
- Concentrate fully on each motion — focus on your body, on lengthening the muscles and maintaining good posture.

Not sure about the moves? Consider a session with a trained Pilates instructor. She can explain the positions and make sure you're using proper form so you don't get injured.

Anti-aging scam is risky business

Have you heard of the "sweet syringe of youth"? A shot of human growth hormone (HGH) and you'll build stronger muscles, rev up your sex drive, lose weight, sleep better, and think more clearly. Or so say the advertisers who tout the miraculous anti-aging properties of this synthetic drug.

But scientists have found little evidence that boosting growth hormones in healthy adults will provide any health benefits, and they could cause harm.

Research on HGH injections discovered they contributed to joint and muscle pain, carpal tunnel syndrome, swelling, numbness and tingling, and possibly even diabetes, heart disease, and cancer. Plus the Food and Drug Administration does not regulate over-the-counter hormones, so you have no guarantee of their safety.

Recent studies have found that, as you age, you're actually better off with less insulin-like growth factor-1 (IGF-1), a compound related to HGH. Lower levels may contribute to a longer life and lower risk of cancer.

Slow and gentle way to better balance

Would you like to try a remarkable, low-impact exercise that relieves dizziness and balance disorders? Set your sights on the ancient Chinese art of tai chi.

Tai chi is a fun and easy way to improve your balance. It teaches you to be aware of your surroundings and helps strengthen your hip muscles, improve your posture, and balance the weight distribution on your legs. Better balance means fewer falls. In fact, studies show tai chi can reduce your risk of falling by almost 50 percent.

Stroke survivors who practiced tai chi experienced fewer falls than those who were not practicing tai chi or participating in another type of fitness program, one study found. And people with mild to moderate Parkinson's disease showed significant improvements in balance after participating in a six-month tai chi program.

The benefits of this amazing workout don't stop there. Tai chi also boosts your memory skills, relieves stress, and relaxes your heart and mind. Plus, it's so helpful in easing arthritis pain and stiffness that it even has its own program designed specifically for arthritis sufferers.

You may have seen tai chi followers in parks or other areas doing a series of postures and slow, continuous movements. These actions make up a "form" or set that helps relax and align your body. A basic short form can have 13 to 40 moves and take between three to 20 minutes to complete.

The workout is fun to do in a class and easy enough to practice alone at home. Look for tai chi classes at local senior centers, community centers, and YMCAs. Keep these tips in mind when you start.

- Wear comfortable shoes and loose clothing.
- Take time to get adjusted to the rhythm of tai chi. You may not be used to moving slowly and gently, so be patient. In a

few weeks, you should start seeing the health benefits you're looking for.

- Control your weight shifts. When you move, first shift all your weight onto your supporting leg. Next, place your other foot, and only then move your weight to that leg. This will help you move smoothly. Remember, tai chi should look fluid — not robotic.
- Stay focused on the move you are in and not the one coming up. Don't move on until you get it right. It's more important to practice tai chi every day than to learn the moves quickly.

5 ways to work out when it's hard to get up

You know exercise can brighten your mood, calm your stress level, and boost your self-esteem. But maybe you're wheelchair bound. Or have a condition like arthritis, obesity, or pulmonary disease that limits your ability to get up and go. But don't just sit there — you can work out with many of the same exercises as your able-bodied friends.

Build strength. You can easily pump iron from a chair by using hand weights, stretchy bands, or even soup cans to build upper body strength. Or use seated exercise machines at a gym to work on your lower body and abdominal muscles.

Work up a sweat. You may not think you can get a cardio workout from a chair, but any series of quick and repetitive movements will raise your heart rate and burn calories. You can do seated aerobics with or without light free weights. Start with something simple, like punching the air with your arms.

Say yes to yoga. Chair yoga is a slower-paced version of the popular Hatha yoga practiced in gyms and yoga studios across the U.S. It's gentle on the body, relieves joint stiffness, and improves flexibility and range of motion. It also promotes deep breathing and relaxation, making it great for stress relief and as a sleep aid, experts say.

Try tai chi. Small, flowing movements make this easy-going form of martial arts popular among people with arthritis. And you can do it in a seated position by performing the movements with your upper body while shifting your lower-body weight to apply pressure to your feet.

Make a splash. Dive into a water therapy program at your local gym or senior center. You can get into a pool with the help of a flotation belt even if you're confined to a chair. Then walk, swim, or just move in the water. You'll build strength and endurance while relieving joint pain and stiffness.

Squeeze your way to lower blood pressure

Got a good golf grip? You may be doing your heart a favor every time you squeeze your club. Scientists have found that regularly grasping and releasing an object like a golf club can lower blood pressure by as much as 10 percent.

Gripping exercises are a form of isometrics, which involve contracting and holding your muscles without moving your joints. You can squeeze anything to strengthen your grip, but the best tool is a spring-loaded device available at sporting goods stores.

Try squeezing for two minutes at a time for a total of 12 to 15 minutes at least three times a week. Your muscles — and your heart — will thank you.

3 no-risk ways to reverse muscle loss

You lose as much as 30 percent of your muscle strength by age 80, health experts say. This process, called sarcopenia, starts in your 40s and 50s when your muscle fibers begin to shrink, become less efficient, and disappear altogether.

Even though sarcopenia mainly shows up in inactive people, even active adults experience some muscle loss. In fact, sarcopenia can do to your muscles what osteoporosis does to your bones. Sarcopenia leads to the weakness, poor coordination, and bad balance, as well as the falls and fractures, that many seniors suffer. But take heart — you have the power to halt your muscle loss and possibly even reverse it. Here's how.

Pump iron. This one solution is the key to maintaining muscle strength. According to the latest research, your strength could jump by an amazing 100 percent if you're a weightlifting senior. Pumping iron works because it encourages your muscles to grow and become more responsive and powerful. A recent study showed that weight training also builds up testosterone in the muscles of older men, which adds to muscle strength and size.

Strengthen your grip. Experts use two measurements to determine if your muscles have weakened — grip strength and decrease in muscle mass. Losing your ability to pinch, hold, or grab things can affect your ability to live independently. Make sure you include isometric hand exercises in your strength training routine. A soft "stress" ball is perfect for toughening your grip.

Eat enough protein. Eating lean red meat along with lifting weights improved the size and strength of muscles in older women, one study found. Researchers recommend eating at least three to four servings a week to keep your body and mind in tiptop condition.

The key is getting enough protein and eating it throughout the day. British researchers found that people who lifted weights but ate less than 70 grams of protein a day had lower muscle mass than expected. But not everyone needs that much. To figure out what's right for you, read *Power up and heal with protein* in the *Protein: the essential body-builder* chapter.

One recent study showed that muscles grew better when people ate a similar amount of protein at each meal rather than getting it all from a big steak dinner. Taking in protein throughout the day gives your body a chance to build and repair muscle continuously.

The bottom line is, your muscles won't stay strong without your help. So work out as hard as your doctor will allow, and fill your diet with high-quality protein, to give your muscles an extra edge as you age.

Arm yourself against brittle bones

Fractures and osteoporosis are turning up in people who were once considered low risk. Find out why this is happening and how you can protect yourself.

What happens. Your skeleton is a newer model than the one you were born with. That's because your body constantly removes sections of old bone and replaces it with new bone made of calcium, phosphorous, and the protein collagen.

Unfortunately, in some people, old bone is removed faster than new bone is made. When that happens, your bones become riddled with holes, like a house losing the mortar between its bricks. Doctors call this problem low bone mineral density (BMD).

BMD that's a little below normal is referred to as osteopenia, while BMD that's worse is osteoporosis. As osteoporosis progresses, bones can become so fragile that a fall can easily fracture your hip, wrist, spine, or other bones.

Are you at risk? Men account for roughly 20 percent of osteoporosis fractures and are twice as likely to die after a hip fracture as women. But older women face the highest odds of osteoporosis and fractures. Why? Women naturally have less bone mass than men, and menopause speeds up bone loss by reducing estrogen levels.

Yet, strangely enough, osteoporosis is increasingly turning up in younger people who:

- take medicines for acid reflux or depression.
- take blood thinning medications or corticosteroids like prednisone.
- have conditions like celiac disease or rheumatoid arthritis.

Your risk of osteoporosis or fractures is also higher if you:

- are white or Asian, especially women.
- have had a long period of not getting enough calcium or vitamin D.
- are a current or former smoker.
- are underweight or have had obesity surgery.
- have low estrogen or testosterone levels.
- don't get enough exercise.
- have type 2 diabetes.
- drink too much alcohol.
- have had a fracture as an adult — or if a parent had a fracture during adulthood.

If you're a man age 70 or older or a woman age 65 or older, ask your doctor about getting screened for osteoporosis. If you haven't reached those ages, but have several of the risk factors listed above, ask your doctor whether you should be screened sooner.

Lower your odds. Take these steps to make your bones more fracture-resistant.

- Sedentary people are more likely to fracture a hip than people who exercise, but you can protect your bones by building muscle. To do this, alternate strength or resistance training with weight-bearing exercises. Strength training includes exercises where you lift your own body weight, lift free weights, or use weight machines or elastic exercise bands.

Good weight-bearing exercises include walking, low-impact aerobics, gardening, or using a stair-climbing machine.

Older adults should also do balance exercises, like tai chi, that strengthen your lower body and sharpen your balance skills.

Get your doctor's permission before starting any new exercise. If you have osteoporosis, check with your doctor to be certain your new exercises and the ones you already do are safe. Some popular exercises, like sit-ups or golfing, may be unsafe for people with osteoporosis because they can raise the risk of spinal fractures.

- Make sure you get enough calcium from foods like dairy products, leafy greens, canned salmon with bones, almonds, and calcium-fortified foods. Women age 50 and older and men age 71 and older need 1,200 milligrams (mg) a day, while men under age 71 should aim for 1,000 mg.
- Aim for 400 to 800 IU of vitamin D every day if you're under age 50, and 800 to 1,000 IU if you're age 50 or older. Good sources include vitamin-D fortified milk and cereal, as well as supplements.
- Limit sodium to 2,300 mg daily — the equivalent of one teaspoon of salt. A Japanese study found that women who ate foods high in sodium had a higher risk of fractures.
- Eat a diet rich in fruits and vegetables. Not only has this been linked to better BMD, but a recent study also suggests the resveratrol in grapes and red wine could increase BMD in men.

Be careful to get enough protein from foods like beans, nuts, seeds, dairy products, and meats. Too little protein has been linked to bone loss, so aim for 46 grams (g) every day if you're a woman and 56 g if you're a man. You can get 31 g from a 5 oz. can of chicken with broth, 13 g from a 1-cup serving of baked beans, 13 g from an 8-oz. serving of plain yogurt, and 16 g from a half cup of tuna salad.

Workout risks: say no to pains and strains

For relief without pills, stop sitting still

You may have heard you should avoid exercise if you have arthritis, but that's not true. Research shows getting more active can help reduce arthritis pain, prevent falls and disability, and improve your walking ability, sleep, and quality of life.

Know your risk factors. Osteoarthritis (OA) is the most common type of arthritis. It strikes your joints and is most common in knees, fingers, hips, spine, and big toes. Every joint is surrounded by cartilage, a slippery cushioning that covers the end of each bone to prevent bones from rubbing together. Over the years, cartilage can gradually wear away, causing arthritis pain. Aging, obesity, family history, joint injuries, and overuse of particular joints may raise your risk.

Fight back with exercise. Movement increases blood flow and nutrients to the cartilage, helping defend against damage and wear. Exercise that strengthens muscle around cartilage also helps. If you already have OA, exercise may reduce pain and stiffness and help prevent a serious disability.

Getting more active can also help you lose weight. Research links a higher body mass index (BMI) with knee, hip, and back pain, but studies suggest losing weight may mean less knee pain and better function.

Make smart choices. The wrong kind of exercise for your arthritis pain and physical condition could make things worse.

For example, vigorous exercise and high-impact, pounding activities such as running put more stress on your joints. Choose low-impact activities like walking instead, and aim for moderate exertion that slightly raises your heart rate and breathing. Experts suggest you also include range-of-motion exercises like stretching, as well as muscle-strengthening exercises.

But check with your doctor before starting an exercise program or a new kind of exercise. You may need professional advice to find an activity that fights pain without causing harm. Your doctor can also tell you when you should rest your painful joints and when you should exercise.

Move away from joint pain. If your doctor gives you permission to exercise, ask him about arthritis-friendly options like these.

- Daily stretching helps lubricate your joints to increase flexibility and range of motion. If needed, relax painful muscles before stretching by applying a heat pack or warm towel for 20 minutes, or reduce swelling by applying an ice pack for 15 minutes. Walk to warm up your muscles before doing 15 minutes of stretching each day. Gently stretch the muscle, and hold the stretch up to 30 seconds without moving. For more details on good stretching, see the *Easy does it: no-work workouts* chapter.

- Take a yoga class. Research shows yoga helps ease arthritis symptoms and the stress that can make arthritis worse.

- Exercise in a pool. You may not walk on water, but walking in water takes some weight — and pain — off your joints. Exercise done in water not only improves mobility, but may be more effective than activity done on land. Ask your doctor or physical therapist where to find a water exercise program, or check for an Arthritis Foundation Aquatic Exercise program at a pool near you. If you have Internet access, visit *www.arthritis.org/programs* to find a class.

- Try walking, especially for knee osteoarthritis. A recent study suggests you can slash your risk of developing problems with walking or climbing stairs by adding 6,000 steps to your day. Start small and gradually build up to that goal. But if you have knee OA, avoid walking in shoes with thick cushioning under the midsole and heel. Those may put more strain on your knees.
- Strength training with light weights three days a week can ease pain and improve range of motion. See the *Stay strong to stop the clock* chapter to learn more about your strength-training options.

For smaller joints, such as those in your hands, feet, ankles, and neck, ask your doctor about more targeted exercises like ankle stretches or wringing out a wet sponge.

When your everyday painkiller turns deadly

When the bumps and bruises of your latest workout have you reaching for a pain pill, stop and take a moment to read the label. You may have already gotten doses of this painkiller from other medicines — and you could be closer to an overdose than you realize.

Acetaminophen (Tylenol) overdose is the leading cause of drug-triggered liver disease and acute liver failure. The Food and Drug Administration (FDA) requires warnings about liver damage on the labels of all over-the-counter (OTC) medicines that contain acetaminophen. Yet acetaminophen overdose sends thousands to hospitals every year. Here's how to protect yourself.

- Acetaminophen is in hundreds of prescription and OTC medicines for colds, flu, fever, sinus problems, allergies, constipation, pain, and sleeping problems. The FDA is eliminating multi-ingredient prescription medicines that contain more than 325 mg of acetaminophen per dose, but

OTC drugs can still have higher doses. You may want to avoid medicines that contain multiple ingredients.

- Before taking any prescription or OTC medicine, check the label to see how much acetaminophen it contains. Acetaminophen may also be called APAP, paracetamol, Acetam, Acetamin, Acetaminop, or Acetaminoph. Don't take more than 3,000 to 4,000 milligrams (mg) in 24 hours, and avoid alcohol while taking this drug. If you have liver disease, a high risk of liver disease, or a history of heavy drinking, ask your doctor whether you can take acetaminophen safely and what your daily limit should be.
- Know the signs of liver damage. Your liver is your body's hazardous materials center, breaking down toxins and cleaning them out of your blood and body. To keep your liver running smoothly, maintain a healthy weight, and avoid taking too much acetaminophen or drinking too much alcohol. Seek medical help if you see signs of liver damage like itching, pale stools, dark urine, a yellowish tinge in your skin or the whites of your eyes, or pain in your upper right midsection.
- Try other remedies for sore muscles and joints like a hot bath, topical menthol creams, heating pads or patches, or ice packs.

8 quick ways to heal your heel pain

You may not think walking can cause that sharp heel pain when you first roll out of bed, but bad walking habits can. Fortunately, a little knowledge may help you ease the pain.

Know your enemy. Severe pain on the underside of your heel can be a sign of plantar fasciitis. The pain happens when overuse or repeated strain causes inflammation of the plantar fascia — the ligament that connects your heel bone to your toes.

Plantar fasciitis is more likely if you wear shoes that fit poorly, have weak arch support, or are worn out. Your risk for this condition may also be higher if you:

- frequently walk on unstable surfaces like sand.
- have flat feet or high arches.
- are overweight.
- have a job that involves a lot of walking and standing on hard surfaces.
- have tight calf muscles that limit the flexibility of your ankles.
- have problems with your walking gait.
- participate in vigorous exercise or sports that injure or put prolonged stress on your feet.

Help yourself heal. Stretching your injured foot should be your top priority. A Scandinavian study found that one exercise is particularly effective at relieving plantar fasciitis.

Position your bare foot on a stair with your heel hanging over the edge and a rolled-up towel under your toes. Grip the stair rail for balance, and bend your other leg so your foot hangs free above the same step. Raise your injured heel slowly enough to count to three, hold still for two seconds, and then slowly lower your heel while counting to three again. Do this stretch 10 to 12 times every other day.

For additional pain relief, try these remedies:

- Soothe the painful spot with ice for 20 minutes three times a day.
- Take anti-inflammatories like aspirin or ibuprofen.
- Wear a nighttime splint that keeps your ankle flexed.

- Rest your overworked feet, and avoid vigorous exercise for a while.
- Cushion your heel with a padded heel cup from the drugstore.
- Wear comfortable shoes, especially those with shock-absorbent cushioning beneath your heel.
- Replace shoes that are worn down or fit poorly.
- Lose weight if you're overweight.

If your heel pain continues despite your best efforts, see your doctor for an accurate diagnosis.

Breaking news: secret weapon beats arthritis misery

Move over, glucosamine supplements. Research suggests a new arthritis pain fighter works better. Although earlier studies suggest glucosamine supplements can fight arthritis pain, several recent studies found they have little or no effect.

Meanwhile, studies of an anti-inflammatory supplement suggest it may relieve arthritis pain as effectively as NSAID painkillers, but with fewer side effects. This supplement is called s-Adenosyl-L-methionone (SAMe). In research trials, people have taken 600 to 1,200 milligrams daily in divided doses.

But check with your doctor before trying any supplement for your arthritis pain. Some supplements may cause dangerous drug interactions when taken with certain prescription or over-the-counter medicines, while others may not be safe for people with particular health conditions. For example, SAMe may be dangerous if you have bipolar disorder or if you take antidepressants or the Parkinson's disease drug levodopa.

Natural way to lower blood pressure 15 points

You want to lower your blood pressure but aren't sure how. Put some pep in your step. Experts say exercising is one of the best ways to lower blood pressure and keep it under control. Plus exercise helps you manage your weight, strengthen your heart, and control stress — all of which contribute to healthy blood pressure.

To lower your pressure, focus on doing aerobic exercise like walking, bicycling, or dancing for 30 to 60 minutes at least three days a week. If you need to, you can break up your exercise into shorter sessions. Regular aerobic exercise can lower your blood pressure from five to 15 points, experts say. In one study, half the people who jogged two miles a day lowered their blood pressure enough that they no longer needed medication.

Resistance exercises like weight training can also lower blood pressure. But for people with high blood pressure, lifting heavy weights can sometimes raise pressure to dangerous levels. Make sure you use light weights and breathe throughout the repetitions to keep your blood pressure steady. Here are a few other precautions you should take.

- Check with your doctor before starting a fitness program. She can tell you if your heart is healthy enough for exercise and give you advice on how much physical activity you can handle.
- If you take a beta blocker, ask your doctor for a stress test. Since beta blockers slow down your heart rate, the test will help you figure out how hard you can push yourself.
- Monitor your heart rate, and make sure you stay within range for your age and health. To lower blood pressure, experts recommend you work out between 50 and 70 percent of your maximum heart rate. This simple formula will help you figure that out. Subtract your age from 220, then multiply your results by .5 and .7. Your heart should beat within this range per minute during exercise. You should be sweating but still able to maintain a conversation.

- Know when to stop. If at any time you feel short of breath, or your heart is beating too fast or irregularly, slow down or rest. And if you feel chest pain, weakness, dizziness, light-headedness, or pressure or pain in your neck, arm, jaw, or shoulder, seek emergency medical help immediately.

Ease your knees with flip-flops and flats

Flip-flops are not athletic shoes. No surprise there. But it is surprising that they can be a good footwear choice if you have bad knees.

Research has found that clogs and stability shoes put more strain on your knees than flip-flops and flat, flexible walking shoes. Stability shoes have a higher heel than other athletic shoes, so choose shoes with flat, flexible soles instead.

Your cheapest option may be flip-flops, but they increase your risk of falls. Avoid them if you have foot or balance problems. Otherwise, wear flip-flops only for short periods, and never wear them to mow the lawn, walk long distances, or play sports. Make a flexible, flat-soled walking shoe your main footwear. Wearing these shoes most of the time may permanently ease the strain on your knees.

Surprise — eat to beat muscle cramps

When a muscle cramp hits, you can try stretching and rubbing the area to work it out. But surprisingly, you have some food choices that can help as well. Try these simple ways to stop muscle cramps and recover from muscle soreness after a workout.

Eat your fruits and veggies. Staying hydrated and keeping your electrolytes in balance may help prevent cramps. Sports drinks can help during a workout, but you can boost their power by eating fruits and vegetables throughout the day. A

German study found that kids who ate the most fruits and vegetables were better hydrated.

That's because foods like strawberries, iceberg lettuce, baby carrots, and grapefruit are all more than 90 percent water. And many water-rich foods are also good sources of electrolytes like magnesium, potassium, calcium, chloride, and even sodium. Try eating broccoli, celery, cucumber, spinach, cantaloupe, bell peppers, and tomatoes to give your body extra water and electrolytes.

Savor sour pickles. Drinking pickle juice to relieve cramps isn't just an old wives tale. A study at North Dakota State University found that drinking 2 1/2 ounces of pickle juice ended cramps 45 percent sooner than drinking nothing. So it's no wonder this remedy is popular among athletes. Some even recommend drinking 2 ounces of pickle juice before a workout to prevent cramps.

Pop some melon balls. Watermelon is the biggest, cheapest fruit you're probably not eating but should be. It's low in calories and high in nutrients, and it might help you recover from muscle soreness. A two-cup serving of watermelon only contains about 90 calories but is high in vitamin A, vitamin C, lycopene, and water.

It also delivers an antioxidant amino acid called citrulline. A recent Spanish study found that drinking citrulline-rich watermelon juice helped reduce muscle soreness better than a placebo. More research is needed to see if eating watermelon provides the same benefits. But remember that watermelon is more than 90 percent water, so enjoying it regularly may help you stay hydrated and prevent cramps.

Try a coconut treat. The American diet is typically low in potassium, so eating more of this mineral may help keep cramps at bay. Bananas and orange juice are good high-potassium choices. But if you're in the mood for a tropical treat, try potassium-rich coconut water, the clear liquid found in coconuts when they're still green. You can buy it at your supermarket, but talk to your doctor first if you take prescription medication to avoid interactions.

Coconut water may have up to five times more potassium than a sports drink for about the same cost, but it has less sodium. If you sweat heavily when you work out, you'll lose a lot of sodium, in which case you're better off rehydrating with a sports drink.

Drink cherry juice. Runners who drank cherry juice daily while training for a 200-mile relay race had less pain after the race, an Oregon study found. Experts think the anthocyanins that give cherries their bright red color also act as anti-inflammatories to fight the inflammation exercise may cause.

If you'd like to try it, look for 100-percent juice made from tart Montmorency cherries at your supermarket or health food store. You can mix it with apple juice if you'd like it sweeter. Drink about two-and-a-half cups of cherry juice each day a week before a strenuous workout as well as the day of the workout itself.

Is it a heart attack — or something else?

You're out exercising when all of a sudden you start wheezing and coughing. Your chest tightens and you feel like you're going to pass out. Don't panic — it's probably not a heart attack. You may have exercise-induced asthma (EIA).

EIA happens when your airways narrow while exercising, making it difficult to take in air. Lots of factors trigger the condition, also called exercise-induced bronchoconstriction. But the most common triggers are cold or dry air, air pollution, high pollen counts, chlorinated swimming pools, and skating rink chemicals.

People with respiratory infections or other lung conditions are more prone to get EIA. And any activity that requires deep breathing for a long period of time — like cycling, running, swimming, and playing soccer — can also trigger it.

Doctors say you should not stop exercising if you get EIA. You just need to do activities that involve short bursts of energy like walking, hiking, ping pong, tennis, and leisurely bike riding. Another good choice is swimming in a heated pool if you can tolerate the chlorine. The warm, moist air makes it easier to breathe. Plus it develops upper body muscles, which can boost your breathing.

Here are some other ideas on how to prevent the misery of exercise-induced asthma.

- **Try fish oil supplements.** Experts say the omega-3 fatty acids in fish oil help keep your airways open by lowering the inflammation that causes asthma. Fish oil may also reduce the need for medication.
- **Take vitamin C.** Studies show this antioxidant helps prevent airways from tightening and increases air flow during exercise.
- **Reduce salt.** Researchers over the years have found low-salt diets fend off asthma. Eating salt seems to make airways constrict.
- **Exercise in the morning.** It's easier on the lungs than in the evening, experts say.
- **Drink caffeine.** It gets a bad rap most of the time, but caffeine helps airways stay free and clear after exercise.
- **Warm up.** Doing 10 minutes of mild to moderate activity before starting your regular exercise routine may help lower the risk of an asthma attack.
- **Breathe through your nose.** You'll help warm and moisten the air before it reaches your lungs.
- **Wear a face mask or scarf.** When you exercise in cold, dry weather, a scarf will help warm and filter the air you breathe.
- **Use an inhaler.** If your doctor recommends it, use an inhaled asthma drug about 10 minutes before exercising.

Step 5: Power up your immune system

Your body's amazing defense system

You might be sitting by yourself reading this right now, but you're not alone. You've got around 100 trillion bacteria cells keeping you company. That's 10 times the number of regular human cells in your body.

Don't freak out. Some of them may be the best friends you'll ever have. Among other things, good bacteria help digest food, destroy organisms that cause disease, metabolize drugs, prevent infection, and provide you with nutrients.

In fact, this "microbiome" — the community of bacteria that live on and in every human being — plays an extremely important role in overall health, impacting conditions like obesity, autism, depression, asthma, and even cancer, a role scientists are just beginning to understand. And while most of the bacteria in your microbiome help you survive by doing things you can't do yourself, there are some bad bugs. They make up less than 1 percent of your bacteria ecosystem, and are probably under attack right now by your very capable defenses — your immune system.

This important network of processes, cells, proteins, tissues, and organs protects you from germs and disease, working hard to form a veritable fortress against invaders that would otherwise make you sick.

The innate immune system. The first line of defense is your innate immune system. Think of it as your body's moat — filled with crocodiles. Its role is to use general strategies to stop germs straight away. It's made up of things like your skin, mucous membranes, and stomach acid. They repel, trap, and destroy many harmful microorganisms before they can cause trouble.

The germs, viruses, parasites, and toxins that make it past your moat face the innate system's roving guard of white blood cells. There are four specialized types — cytokines, natural killer (NK) cells, macrophages, and dendritic cells.

These sound a general alarm and attempt to kill off the intruders. At this point, local inflammation sets in as part of your defense. More blood is directed to the area, and blood vessels widen to accommodate the increased traffic of immune system cells.

In most cases, you never know how hard your body is working to keep you safe. In other instances, you actually experience symptoms — the swelling around a cut or the redness and itching from a mosquito bite, for instance. These are signs of your immune system at work.

The adaptive immune system. When bacteria evade or overcome both levels of your innate system, your second line of defense is called into action — your adaptive immune system. It includes lymph nodes, bone marrow, your spleen, and your thymus. All of these play important roles in producing, storing, and transporting white blood cells.

Just as its name implies, the adaptive system analyzes a specific threat and tailors its reaction accordingly. Much like a police force sends out a traffic cop, a SWAT team, or a homicide detective, depending on the crime, your adaptive system sends out T cells, a type of white blood cell that can be customized to fight a particular infection.

Once the germ is destroyed, these T cells remain in your body for decades, remembering what the germ looked like and how to vanquish it. That is how you build up immunity to various germs.

As you might suppose, your adaptive immunity is constantly evolving as you're exposed to various germs, diseases, and vaccines.

The chink in your armor. Every person's immune system is different. And yours will change throughout your lifetime. When you are young and healthy, you can crank out countless T cells, fighting infection and building immunity against a host of germs. As you age, your body makes fewer and fewer T cells. So when you're faced with a new threat, you have fewer weapons in your arsenal.

In addition, some people have an immune system that works splendidly all the time, fighting infections and disease like a true super trooper. Others have a system that misfires occasionally. For instance, if you suffer from a grass, mold, pet, or food allergy, your immune system is overreacting to harmless materials. Your sneezing, runny nose, hives, or other symptoms are a result of a misguided immune system attack.

And in some cases the immune system utterly fails. It can mistakenly attack healthy cells and organs in your body, causing devastating illnesses like type 1 diabetes, lupus, rheumatoid arthritis, and others. These are called autoimmune diseases.

The amazing protection system in your body, known as your immune system, fends off a constant flood of germs, viruses, and other microscopic villains. Without it, no one would live very long. Most of the time, it does its job efficiently and silently, so it's easy to take it for granted. Don't. Read on to find out what you can do to keep your immune system active and strong.

Get smart about fighting germs

Win the fight against infections

They're lurking all around you, waiting for their chance to attack — viruses, bacteria, fungi, and other foreign invaders. A healthy immune system has no problem shutting them out, but one that's starved for zinc, vitamin D, and other nutrients might. Good nutrition can make all the difference in battling an illness, especially as you get older.

Viruses and bacteria are behind most infections. Viruses can cause colds, coughs, sore throats, and the flu. Bacteria, on the other hand, bear the blame for strep throat, urinary tract infections, tuberculosis, and most ear infections. Both types of bugs make you sick, but they do it in completely different ways.

- Viruses break into your body's cells and take over. They hijack the cells' machinery to churn out more viruses, which then infect more cells.
- Most bacteria in your body are actually beneficial, but about one in eight can make you sick. Some attack specific areas. Others, like *E. coli*, pump out toxins that make you ill. And still others multiply so much they clog your blood vessels or hinder your heart.

Fungi and parasites are no slouches either when it comes to causing problems. Fungi lead to yeast infections, thrush, athlete's foot, and ringworm, while organisms called parasites cause malaria and giardia, among others.

It can take your body days or weeks to fight off a germ. But the more times your immune system encounters the same bug, the faster it will defeat it in the future.

What you eat matters, too, especially as you get older. Poor nutrition makes you more susceptible to infections. Then your body drains what nutrients it does have to fight the illness, leaving you even more depleted and vulnerable. Older adults are more likely to suffer from nutritional deficiencies, which may partly explain why your immune system weakens with age.

The good news — you can reverse this downward slide by eating better. In one recent study, scientists followed three groups of seniors for six months.

- One group focused on eating better. They made sure to eat five servings of fruits and vegetables each day, fish twice a week, nuts once a week, and only whole-grain breads and cereals.
- Another group took a daily supplement of zinc, beta carotene, selenium, and vitamins E and C containing nutrients in amounts similar to what the food group was getting.
- A third group took a daily placebo, a fake pill that looked exactly like the supplement.

Seniors in the food and supplement groups came down with the same number of infections as those in the placebo group, but their illnesses didn't last as long or impact their life as much. The food group faired best of all. They suffered fewest weeks of illness and made the fewest sick-visits to the doctor and hospital.

These seniors are onto something. Certain nutrients play key roles in your immune system. Without them, it can't fend off illnesses as effectively — sort of like boxing with one hand tied behind your back. Get smart. Pack your body with super nutrients proven to improve your immune system and keep you well.

Zinc. A zinc deficiency could make you more vulnerable to infections, prevent immune cells from doing their jobs properly, and create runaway inflammation. When your immune system spots an invading germ, it starts pumping zinc from your bloodstream into white blood cells known as monocytes. All this zinc protects them from the inflammation they produce while fighting germs. Without enough, the monocytes will die.

Your body naturally absorbs less zinc with age, which contributes to growing inflammation and a weakening immune system. On top of that, you probably don't eat enough of it. Two out of five elderly Americans get too little zinc in their diets. Oysters, red meat, and fortified breakfast cereals are top sources.

A mineral that can spell trouble

Some experts suggest taking a daily vitamin and mineral supplement that contains the Recommended Dietary Allowance (RDA) of zinc — but don't take large amounts of zinc by itself. Excess zinc actually suppresses immune function and may block your body from absorbing other important nutrients, like iron and copper.

Vitamin D. Experts long ago realized that sunlight, which triggers your skin to make vitamin D, helped people fight tuberculosis. So it stands to reason that a shortage could make you sicker. Case in point — Native Americans have extremely high rates of vitamin D deficiency. They are also six times more likely to die from tuberculosis than other Americans. This vital nutrient helps your immune system:

- produce macrophages, white blood cells that literally eat and destroy disease-causing germs.
- crank out killer T cells, which destroy germs, and regulatory T cells, which keep inflammation under control.

- grow and maintain B cells, immune cells that tell your body which microbes to attack.

Native Americans aren't the only ones who typically need more vitamin D. If you are elderly, dark-skinned, overweight, obese, or living in the northern U.S. or Canada, you may be deficient. Ask your doctor to test your blood levels. He can prescribe potent supplements, if needed. Try to spend a few minutes in the sunshine each day. As little as five minutes can do you good. And add more vitamin D to your diet with foods such as salmon, trout, milk, and fortified cereal.

Fruits add punch to vitamin D

Go ahead, add a few blueberries to your yogurt. Blueberries and red grapes may multiply vitamin D's impact on your immune system. Both fruits contain stilbenoids, compounds that plants produce to protect themselves from infections. Vitamin D bolsters your innate immune system, the body's first line of defense against infections. Now a new study shows that stilbenoids partner with vitamin D, making it several times more effective.

These results came from a lab study. Scientists don't know how many of the stilbenoids in food actually make it into your bloodstream. Still, these fruits boast many other health benefits, so go ahead and enjoy. You may make your immune system very happy.

Vitamin A. Your ability to fend off infections relies heavily on having enough vitamin A in your body, since it helps keep the barriers of your innate immune system healthy. Not surprisingly, vitamin A deficiency impairs your immunity and makes you more likely to catch infectious diseases. Measles, for example, is more severe in children who are vitamin A-deficient.

Eating liver is the quickest way to get a shot of vitamin A. Don't make a habit of it, however. This nutrient can be toxic in large amounts. Milk and fortified cereals are safe, everyday sources. In plants, vitamin A is formed from beta carotene. Sweet potatoes, carrots, and spinach are super sources of beta carotene.

Vitamin B6. Certain chronic illnesses, like heart disease, drain your body's stores of B6. That, in turn, depresses your immune system. It needs this vitamin to make T and B cells, as well as substances that stop your immune response from spiraling out of control. Like vitamin A, too much B6 can be toxic, so only take supplements if your doctor recommends them. Otherwise, focus on food sources like yellowfin tuna, beef liver, fortified cereals, baked potato with skin, and enriched rice.

PUFAs. EPA and DHA, two polyunsaturated fatty acids (PUFAs), are woven into the walls of your immune cells. They control the messages these cells send and receive. When your immune system responds to an invading germ, it uses PUFAs to call for backup. Past research found that the PUFAs in fish and fish oil helped cut the number of infections, including pneumonia, people caught and shortened their duration. DHA seems to be particularly important for B cell functioning.

Cold-water fish such as salmon, sardines, trout, and herring are excellent sources of EPA and DHA. Your body can also turn linolenic acid, another fat, into EPA and DHA as needed. For more linolenic acid, cook with canola oil, drizzle flaxseed or wheat germ oil on your salad, and add walnuts to your morning oatmeal.

Vitamin E. This nutrient protects the fragile PUFAs in your immune cells from getting damaged during the fight against germs. It may also offset age-related slumps in immune function. In one study, taking 200 international units (IU) of synthetic vitamin E daily strengthened elderly people's immune systems and lowered their risks of catching colds and other infections.

Talk to your doctor before trying supplements. They can increase your risk of bleeding, a dangerous side effect if you already take blood-thinning drugs. Food sources, on the other hand, are perfectly safe. Raw (uncooked) oils such as safflower, wheat germ, and canola are loaded with it. So are dry roasted sunflower seeds, salad dressing, mayonnaise made with safflower oil, and fortified cereals.

Selenium. The major organs in your immune system, including your spleen and lymph nodes, are jam-packed with selenium. This mineral boosts the activity of T cells and white blood cells. Selenium deficiency not only puts your body under stress — it also causes viruses to mutate and become more severe.

Increasing your daily dose of selenium can aid your immunity even if you aren't technically deficient. Megadoses of selenium can be toxic, so stick with food. Canned tuna, salmon, shellfish, pork, and other meats are top-notch natural sources.

Surprising new culprit in sinus misery

Health problems like year-round allergies, diabetes, and gastroesophageal reflux disease (GERD) make you more susceptible to chronic sinusitis (CRS), but new research suggests your own immune system is sometimes to blame.

Scientists took samples of the bacteria and fungi living in the sinuses of healthy people and in those with CRS. Surprisingly, the healthy group harbored the same bugs in their sinuses as did people with chronic sinusitis. The difference — the CRS-sufferers had much more inflammation.

That leads experts to think some people develop CRS because their immune systems needlessly attack the harmless microbes that naturally live in their sinuses. This overreaction creates an endless cycle of inflammation, leading to chronic sinusitis.

How your body wages war on germs

A healthy immune system is like a carefully orchestrated battle plan, with different cells working together to capture, destroy, and clean up foreign invaders.

Germs that enter your body are first spotted by granulocytes, a type of immune cell that kills germs by eating them. A few sneak past and travel deeper into your body, where they attack or infect healthy cells. That's where dendritic cells step in. These specialized immune cells hang out among your body's other cells looking for intruders. When they find one, they grab it with their long arms and eat it.

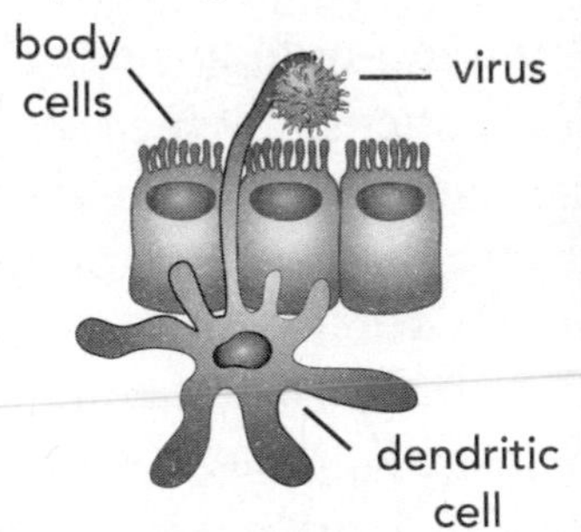

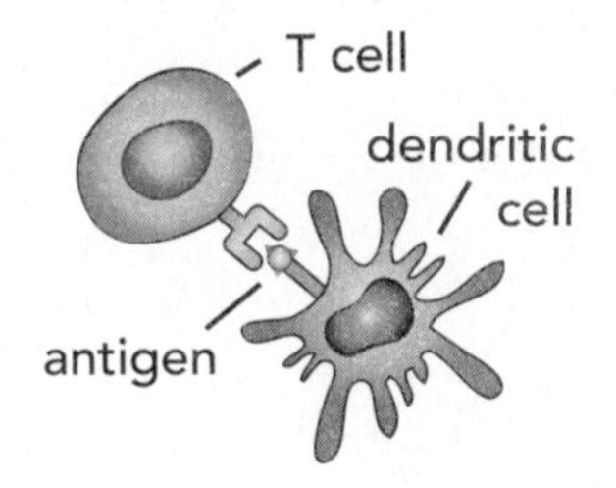

They digest the germ and display a tiny piece of it, called an antigen, on their surfaces. Antigens are like a criminal's mug shot. The dendritic cells travel to the nearest lymph node and show it to the T and B cells stationed there.

Eventually, one of the T cells will recognize that germ's antigen from a past infection. This T cell will "turn on," multiplying itself and turning on B cells and other T cells. Some B cells turn into plasma B cells, while others turn into memory B cells.

Plasma B cells leave the lymph node and travel to where the germs were spotted. They shoot out substances called antibodies that lock onto germs and infected cells. Antibodies prevent the germ from invading other cells and mark it for destruction. Killer T cells shoot infected cells, blowing them to pieces. Then nearby macrophages eat the pieces and clean up the mess.

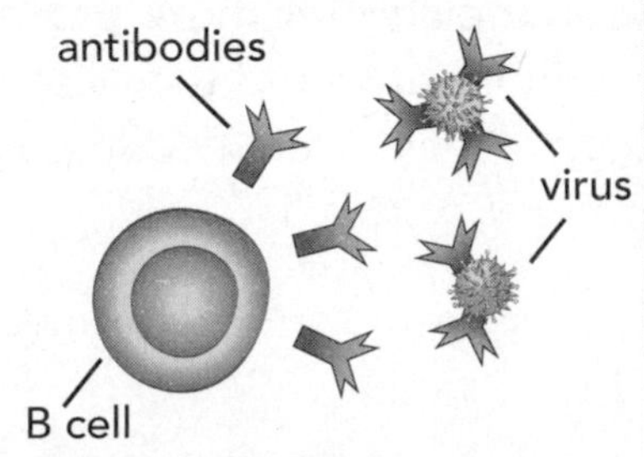

Proven tactics for fighting off infections

They're everywhere — supplements that claim to enhance your immunity and even prevent the common cold. Sounds great, but the science behind them doesn't hold up. One in five makes illegal claims about treating or preventing an illness. Don't waste precious money on products that may not work. Bolster your body's defenses for free.

Get good-quality sleep. You might as well call it vitamin Z. Study after study suggests that a lack of sleep hurts your ability to fight infections. Getting six or fewer hours of sleep a night changes how your immune system responds to germs. In fact, people who routinely slept less than five hours a night were more likely to develop pneumonia in one study. Quality matters, too. People who slept poorly or not enough were more likely to catch colds in another study. While you sleep, your immune system:

- moves immune cells from your bloodstream into lymph nodes, where they enlist T and B cells to fight germs.
- produces more T and B cells and attacks foreign invaders.
- reinforces its memory of germs that it fought in the past.

Sleep loss ramps up your sympathetic nervous system. This squashes your body's virus-fighting response and stimulates unhealthy inflammation. Of course, nabbing enough z's isn't always easy. Smooth your journey into dreamland with help from the stories *Take these smart steps to sounder sleep* and *Target sleep problems with better nutrition* in the *Sleep right to save your life* chapter.

Keep moving for more protection. Bodies in motion tend to stay in motion, and they also tend to stay healthy. Moderate exercise may actually reverse age-related changes in your immune system by:

- increasing your resistance to upper respiratory infections.

- helping T cells multiply and preventing their breakdown as they age.
- releasing endorphins, which increase the number of natural killer cells in your body.
- lowering your cortisol levels, a stress hormone that suppresses your immune system.

It shows. People who are active on a regular basis get fewer infections than those who spend most of their time sitting. And it doesn't take much. The American College of Sports Medicine recommends exercising for 150 minutes each week. That could simply mean walking your dog for 30 minutes a day, five days a week.

Consider trying tai chi or yoga, as well. Older adults who took tai chi for 15 weeks saw a boost in their immunity, specifically against the shingles virus. Yoga impacts your immune system almost immediately, within two hours of practicing.

Curb those vices. Drinking alcohol in moderation may improve your immune response to infections, but heavy drinking does the opposite. Moderation means one or two drinks a day for men and one drink a day for women. A drink is equal to one 5-ounce glass of wine or 12 ounces of beer. But if you don't drink, don't start.

Smoking poses other problems. It encourages your body to kill the beneficial bacteria that live in your mouth. These harmless bugs normally crowd out the bad ones, but when they die, disease-causing bacteria move in and take over. It's one more reason to kick the habit.

5 stress-busting steps to help you stay well

Long-term stress may be your body's worst enemy. Short-term stress ramps up your immune system, but chronic stress suppresses it. It causes your brain to release small, but steady, amounts of glucocorticoid hormones, which block monocytes, macrophages, natural killer cells, and T cells from doing their jobs, and prevent your body from making memory immune cells after an infection. Stress could even help cancer spread to other parts of your body.

Surprisingly, social and emotional stress can harm your immunity more than physical stress. Loneliness, isolation, divorce, problems at work or in relationships, and caring for an ill loved one are all examples of social stress. Everyone faces these challenges at some point. How you handle them could make the difference in staying healthy.

- Caregivers, cut yourself some slack. Seniors looking after loved ones have higher levels of the stress hormone cortisol, and fewer antibodies for fending off the flu virus. You can't give care if you get sick. Call United Way by dialing 211. It can help you find nearby respite services.

- Stay in touch with your friends, and ask for help when you need it. Of people caring for a spouse with Alzheimer's disease, those with the fewest friends and the least amount of help saw the biggest drop in T cell function, a major marker of immune health.

- Force yourself to be social, especially after a loss. Your body reacts to loneliness the same as it does chronic stress. People who are lonely have more dormant viruses and inflammation-causing compounds in their bodies — all signs of a weakened immune system.

- Seek marriage counseling if you need it. In one study, spouses who worried the most about their relationships had higher cortisol levels and fewer T cells. Cortisol keeps your body from making T cells, which, in turn, hampers your immune response to germs.

- Put your feelings on paper. In a study of people with a life-threatening virus, those who journaled about their emotions, both good and bad, stayed well longer.

Can't-miss action plan to combat colds

Your immune system is incredible, but germs, like the ones that cause colds, can change fast. They're like criminals who don a new disguise every time they rob a bank, making it harder for the cops to catch them. Eventually, your immune system will recognize the germs and fight back, but that will take time.

To make matters more difficult, colds aren't caused by just one virus. The rhinovirus is the most common cause, but it comes in more than 100 different varieties. At least 100 other viruses also cause colds. No wonder scientists haven't been able to find a cure.

The good news is, you generally catch fewer colds as you age. It's one of the benefits of getting older. Improve your odds even further with some smart preventive measures.

Take commonsense precautions. A look at 67 studies shows that washing your hands frequently is the surest way to avoid catching a cold, especially if you spend time around children. No need to buy fancy, antibacterial soaps, either. Research has found they work no better than regular soap.

Skip the alcohol-based hand sanitizers and use a foaming one made with benzalkonium chloride, instead. It leaves a residue on your hands that protects against cold viruses.

Increase your vitamin D. Vitamin C helps prevent colds in extreme athletes, like marathon runners, but it won't do a thing for the average person. Vitamin D might. Research links low levels of vitamin D in your blood with a higher risk of respiratory infections. In a Swedish study, people who were prone to respiratory tract infections took daily vitamin D supplements for a year, and cut their risk of infection by 23 percent. Supplements probably won't help people whose vitamin D levels are normal. Ask your doctor to check yours, especially if you are prone to long-lasting colds and respiratory infections.

No matter how careful you are, you will eventually come down with a cold. It will last seven to 10 days, on average, but some poor souls can suffer for up to three weeks. Don't be one of them. Shorten your cold and relieve your symptoms with these remedies.

Zinc lozenges. Start sucking on these within 24 hours of your first symptoms, and they could shorten your cold by two to three days and make your symptoms milder. Scientists think that holding a zinc lozenge in your mouth keeps the cold virus from multiplying. Keep in mind they may cause nausea in some people and leave a bad taste in your mouth.

Ask your doctor if they are safe for you to take. Those made with zinc acetate work better than those with zinc sulfate. Follow the dosage instructions, but take enough to get at least 75 milligrams of zinc each day. And avoid lozenges that contain citric or tartaric acid, flavorings that may make them less effective.

Andrographis. Supplements made with this Asian shrub may shorten a cold and ease the sore throat, drainage, and earache that come with it. People in one successful study took Kalmcold, a supplement that contains andrographis. Check ingredient labels for this herb, or buy an extract containing 5 percent andrographolide.

It's not safe for everyone. Avoid it if you have diabetes, a bleeding disorder, high or low blood pressure, or take blood-thinning medications.

Echinacea purpurea. Start taking this supplement as soon as you come down with a cold, and you could ease your symptoms and end it faster. It specifically improved runny noses, sore throats, sneezing, and fatigue in one study. Look for capsules or liquids that contain the above-ground parts of the plant — the leaves, stem, and flowers — not the root. And be sure to buy *Echinacea purpurea*, not *Echinacea angustifolia*. The latter is useless against colds.

Do-it-yourself relief from sinus infections

Sinusitis — everyone has it at some point, but chances are you and your doctor are both treating it all wrong. Antibiotics are unlikely to help, and decongestants can actually make it worse. The best relief comes from simple, at-home treatments you can do yourself.

Sinusitis is really just inflammation of your sinuses and nasal passages. The membrane lining your sinuses produces mucus, which normally flows out through your nose. When something irritates that membrane, like a cold virus, allergies, cigarette smoke, or bacteria, it swells. The swelling blocks the exit route to your nose, trapping air and mucus in your sinuses. As the mucus gets thicker, bacteria may start to flourish, setting the stage for a secondary infection.

Doctors classify sinusitis by how long it lasts — acute lasts fewer than four weeks, subacute between four and 12 weeks, and chronic more than 12 weeks. If you have more than three episodes in one year, you have recurrent sinusitis.

Is it viral or bacterial? Viruses, including the cold virus, cause up to 98 percent of sinusitis. Less than 2 percent of those cases go on to develop a secondary bacterial infection. That means bacteria play a role only about 4 percent of the time. The other 96 percent of the time, antibiotics won't help.

Both viral and bacterial sinusitis have similar symptoms — including colored mucus, coughing, and congestion — so they can be hard to tell apart. But if your symptoms match one of these three patterns, you may well have a bacterial infection.

- They last more than 10 days with no improvement.
- You have severe symptoms or a fever of 102 degrees, accompanied by colored mucus or facial pain lasting at least three days in a row.
- Your sinus symptoms fade as you recover from a cold, then suddenly become worse, possibly with a new fever, headaches, or more mucus.

Sinusitis goes away on its own in seven out of 10 people, although you may need antibiotics to get over a bacterial infection. Here's how to help your body heal faster, no matter what caused your sinusitis.

Get steamed up. Lean over a bowl of hot, not boiling, water, cover your head with a towel to trap the steam, and inhale for 10 minutes. Do this up to four times a day.

Drink more. Drinking fluids, especially water, helps lubricate swollen mucous membranes. A cup of hot tea or bowl of soup packs a one-two punch of liquid and steam.

Wash it away. Rinsing your nasal and sinus passages several times a day can help clear out mucus. Make a saline rinse with 1 teaspoon of Kosher or sea salt; 2 cups of warm water, either distilled or boiled for three minutes; and a pinch of baking soda.

Rethink meds. Decongestants can worsen sinus inflammation, and research suggests they don't help treat sinusitis. Don't turn to antihistamines, either. They dry mucus so it can't drain out. Check the labels on over-the-counter cold and allergy remedies. Many contain antihistamines.

Of course, the best way to treat sinusitis is to avoid getting it in the first place. Since respiratory viruses are a major cause, practice good hygiene habits during cold season, and be sure to get your annual flu vaccine. Air pollutants can trigger sinus swelling, too, so quit smoking and don't use strong-smelling chemicals while cleaning. Keep your nose and sinus membranes moist with sterile saline sprays and rinses, as needed. Use a humidifier to moisten dry, indoor air in winter.

Startling causes of chronic cough

Coughing that lingers after an upper respiratory tract infection should go away on its own, but see your doctor if your cough lasts more than eight weeks. It could be a sign of other problems.

- Half of asthma sufferers have cough-variant asthma, where a cough — not shortness of breath — is their only symptom.
- Not everyone with gastroesophageal reflux disease (GERD) feels heartburn. Some people suffer from "silent" reflux. Acid irritating your respiratory tract could cause you to cough.
- As many as one in five people taking ACE inhibitors for high blood pressure experience chronic coughing as a side effect. It typically starts within six weeks of beginning the drug.
- The vagus nerve controls both constipation and coughing, which could explain why elderly adults with constipation may also cough. Constipation can also cause GERD and, hence, a cough.
- Uncontrolled diabetes can lead to nerve damage, or neuropathy, in your voice box, which can trigger coughing.

Give the slip to antibiotic side effects

Antibiotics are not cure-alls. They can't treat viral infections like the flu, for instance, and they can trigger serious side effects and drug interactions. Protect yourself from the downsides with this advice.

Try probiotics. Antibiotics often cause diarrhea because they kill the good gut bugs keeping you healthy, while killing the bad bacteria making you ill. These good bacteria normally prevent the bad ones, like *Clostridium difficile*, from taking root in your intestines. Without them, *C. diff* can flourish, causing diarrhea, an inflamed colon, and even death.

Research shows taking probiotics while on antibiotics can reduce your risk of diarrhea by nearly two-thirds. Look for foods and supplements that contain the bacteria *Lactobacillus rhamnosus GG*, *Lactobacillus paracasei*, or *Saccharomyces boulardii*. Take them at least two hours after your antibiotic for the greatest effect.

Beware interactions. Common drugs don't mix with certain antibiotics. Talk with your doctor about avoiding these combinations:

- the antibiotics clarithromycin or erythromycin with statin medications for high cholesterol. The combination can lead to muscle damage, kidney damage, or death.
- clarithromycin or erythromycin with calcium-channel blockers for high blood pressure, particularly nifedipine. The mix could cause a dangerous drop in blood pressure, leading to shock or kidney damage.
- clarithromycin, ciprofloxacin, or sulfamethoxazole-trimethoprim with the diabetes drugs glipizide or glyburide. The combination could trigger a dangerous drop in blood sugar, especially in women and the elderly.

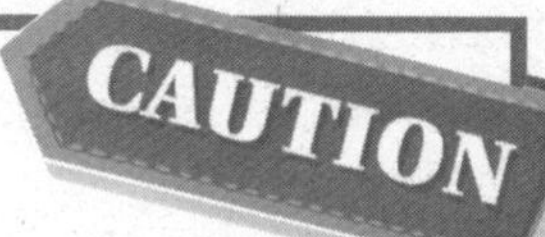

Dodge hidden danger in sinus rinse

The very water you use to rinse your sinuses may actually be causing your sinus infections. Doctors sampled the germs living in the sinuses of people with chronic sinusitis, then sampled the tap water in their homes. Half had the same tough-to-kill bacteria in their sinuses as in their faucets, showers, and water filters. They had been rinsing their sinuses with water straight from those taps and filters.

Never use tap water as a sinus rinse, unless you boil it first for at least three minutes, then let it cool. Filters are no guarantee, either, since several people in this study had bacteria growing in their water filters. Use sterile water, available by prescription at your pharmacy. Or, if that's too expensive, buy distilled water at the store.

6 easy actions to defeat the flu

The flu virus can do more than make you sick for a few days, especially if you're over the age of 65. "No one should confuse influenza with a minor illness," warns Gregory Poland, Professor of Medicine at the Mayo Clinic. As many as 49,000 people die from it each year.

The hallmark headache, fever, muscle aches, chills, cough, sore throat, and weakness generally last two to seven days. Most people recover fine and go on with their lives. But the flu strikes some people — including seniors — particularly hard, causing serious illness, hospitalization, and death. "All human immune systems weaken with age, so when older people get the flu and get knocked down further, they are more likely to get other infections, such as pneumonia," explains Andrew Duxbury, associate professor at the University of Alabama School of Medicine.

Even basic flu symptoms can permanently change the life of an elderly person. "Just being knocked into bed for as little as three or four days can, in a very frail older person, affect their ability to walk and do for themselves," says Duxbury. "It can cause a spiral in disabilities and increase chances of falls and injuries."

Get a flu shot. According to the Centers for Disease Control and Prevention (CDC), all adults should get the flu vaccine each year, unless their doctor says otherwise. It protects you from more than the flu. It also lowers your risk of heart attack and hospitalization. Flu shots are critical for people over the age of 65, or who have asthma, lung disease, or a chronic illness such as heart disease, diabetes, or cancer.

Don't rush to get it in July. Wait until September or October. Flu season runs from late fall to early spring, peaking in January or February. The vaccine protects you for six to eight months. Getting it too early could leave you vulnerable toward the end of the season.

- Ask your doctor about the new quadrivalent vaccine. It protects against four strains of flu, rather than the three strains in other flu shots.
- Ask about the new high-dose vaccine if you are over age 65. It's four times stronger than the regular shot and may offer seniors better protection from the flu.

Stop the spread. The flu spreads mainly when an infected person coughs, sneezes, or talks; and when you touch a surface like a doorknob that has flu virus on it, then touch your mouth, eyes, or nose.

- Try to stay at least 6 feet away from sick people. The virus can travel that far when an infected person sneezes.
- The flu virus can survive on your fingers for up to 30 minutes, so wash your hands often with soap and warm water. Use alcohol-based hand sanitizers when soap isn't available.
- Wipe down surfaces such as doorknobs and mobile phones. A damp, microfiber cloth removes germs from smooth surfaces like a cellphone. Bleach kills the virus better than rubbing alcohol, but don't use it on electronic devices.

Raise the humidity. Flu virus spreads more easily in dry air. That may explain why flu season peaks during the driest winter months and strikes harder in particularly dry winters. Keeping the humidity above 40 percent helps kill the virus quickly.

What happens if you get the flu? These steps can help you bounce back.

Seek help. Head to the clinic or doctor's office as soon as flu symptoms hit. Taking antiviral drugs within 48 hours of developing the flu reduces your risk of ending up in the hospital or dying.

Stay hydrated. Elderly people, in particular, should drink plenty of fluids. They have a duller sense of thirst and can become dehydrated in less than one day with the flu. Water is a great option, but 100-percent cranberry juice could help, too. People who drank two glasses a day had less-severe flu symptoms in one study. Scientists think the colorful compounds in cranberries may strengthen the front-line immune cells fighting the virus.

Rest up. Your body needs to focus all of its energy on fighting the flu, so take it easy. That said, the elderly should sit up in bed a bit and even move around a little to keep their lungs healthy and prevent pneumonia from setting in.

Block flu from becoming pneumonia

Catching the flu can open the door for pneumonia, especially in seniors and smokers. While your immune system is busy fighting off the flu virus, it dials back on destroying bacteria. This can allow them to gain a foothold in your lungs.

The one-two punch of flu and pneumonia can be deadly. It's what killed most people during the Spanish Flu epidemic between 1918 and 1920. Guard yourself by getting vaccinated. Experts now recommend everyone over age 65 get two different pneumonia vaccines instead of one for maximum protection.

If you have never received a pneumonia vaccine, your doctor will give you Prevnar 13 first, followed by Pneumovax 23 six to 12 months later. If you received a single pneumonia vaccine in the past, it was probably Pneumovax 23. Ask your doctor about beefing up your protection with the new shot, Prevnar 13.

Sure-fire way to cure most ulcers

Stomach ulcers have two main causes, and neither one is spicy food or stress. A common bacterium, *Helicobacter pylori*, causes more than half of all stomach ulcers. It eats away at the mucous lining that protects the stomach from its own acid. The acid then damages the tissue underneath, creating an ulcer.

Certain medicines, including Fosamax and nonsteroidal anti-inflammatory drugs (NSAIDs), such as aspirin and ibuprofen, can also damage the stomach lining and cause ulcers, particularly if you have an *H. pylori* infection.

The good news is, killing the bacterium can cure your ulcer. Your doctor will test you for *H. pylori* and, if you have it, prescribe antibiotics and acid-suppressing drugs. Eight out of 10 times, this works. Research suggests adding these supplements to your drug regimen can make success more likely. Ask your doctor if they could help you.

- a probiotic containing the bacteria *Lactobacillus rhamnosus GG*, *Bifidobacterium*, or *Saccharomyces boulardii*.
- 500 milligrams of vitamin C plus 200 IU of vitamin E, twice a day.

Also, quit smoking, and avoid NSAIDs and alcohol. These worsen ulcers and prevent them from healing.

Say 'goodbye' to shingles for good

Shingles sounds harmless enough. It's just a rash, right? Wrong. The rash may fade in a few weeks, but the intense pain can linger for years. What's more, the illness dramatically increases your risk of stroke. Thanks to modern medicine, you don't have to be a victim.

The infection strikes when the same virus that gave you chickenpox as a child "wakes up" again in your body. The varicella-zoster, or chickenpox, virus lays dormant in your nerves for years. It can suddenly surge to life again, causing the rash and pain known as shingles. Anyone who has had chickenpox can get it, including children, but it's most likely to strike if you:

- are over age 60.
- have a weak immune system.
- take immune-suppressing drugs.
- have cancer.
- take steroids or chemotherapy.
- have an autoimmune disorder, such as rheumatoid arthritis.
- have chronic lung or kidney disease.

The Centers for Disease Control and Prevention (CDC) says you have a 30 percent chance of developing it during your life. Most people only get shingles once, but it can hit two or even three times.

You will probably notice a burning, tingling pain at first, followed by a rash that forms blisters. Like chickenpox, you can spread shingles to other people. "You are contagious as long as you have blisters and ulcers," explains Khalilah Babino, an immediate care doctor at Loyola University Health System. "Since it can be spread from person to person, it is important to cover your rash and wash your hands frequently."

Most of the time, the rash develops around your chest or abdomen, but it can appear on your arms, legs, or face, which is particularly dangerous. "If you develop shingles on your face, especially near your eye, you should seek immediate medical care as this type may result in loss of vision," Babino warns.

Long-lasting side effects. The rash will eventually fade, but the pain may linger for months or years. The virus drills tiny holes in your nerves to infect them, damaging them in the process. These nerves carry electrical signals that leak out through the holes, making the nerves misfire painfully. It's called postherpetic neuralgia (PHN). Only one in six people develop PHN, but the older you are when you get shingles, the higher your risk and the more severe the pain will be.

Surprisingly, shingles raises your risk of stroke for six months after the illness, especially if the rash spread to your eyes. The first month is the most dangerous. You are 63 percent more likely to have a stroke then.

An ounce of prevention. Avoid these problems by getting the zoster vaccine. It slashes your shingles risk by half. It also cuts your risk of PHN by two-thirds if you develop shingles.

The CDC recommends that everyone over age 60 get it, unless you have a weakened immune system or take biologic drugs for rheumatoid arthritis. Doctors can give it to adults as young as age 50. You can even get it if you have already had shingles, to prevent another outbreak.

A pound of cure. See your doctor immediately if you suspect you have shingles. Taking an anti-viral drug within three days of developing symptoms, preferably before blisters form, can ease the pain and shorten the illness. "The medication does not kill the virus, like antibiotics kill bacteria, but they help slow the virus and speed recovery," explains Babino. "The earlier these medications are started, the more effective they are against the virus." Anti-viral drugs can also reduce your stroke risk following a bout of shingles. But you may have to ask for them. Doctors in one study only prescribed anti-virals to half of people suffering from shingles.

Ask around for shingles vaccine

Not all doctors' offices keep the shingles vaccine on hand. If yours doesn't, ask your pharmacist or local health clinic if they carry it. Remember to tell your doctor if you get vaccinated elsewhere, so she can note it in your file.

Pump up vaccines' protection

Thanks to vaccines, people no longer end up crippled by polio or dead from smallpox. They work by teaching your immune system to recognize and fight a specific virus or bacteria.

You aren't done with them once you leave childhood. The Centers for Disease Control and Prevention (CDC) recommends these vaccines for adults, with one exception — people with weakened immune systems should not get vaccines for shingles or chickenpox.

Age	Vaccine
all adults	annual flu shot
50 years and older	tetanus/diphtheria booster every 10 years, one-time chickenpox vaccine if you have not had chickenpox
60 years and older	one-time zoster (shingles) vaccine
65 years and older	one-time, two-dose pneumonia vaccine

Many vaccines don't protect seniors as well as they do children. Your immune system needs special "naïve" T cells to learn how to fight new germs. Unfortunately, your body produces fewer and fewer with age. Never fear. These tricks can make vaccines more effective.

- Sleep seven or more hours a night. The hepatitis B vaccine didn't protect as well in people who slept less.
- Eat at least five servings of fruits and vegetables daily. Seniors who went from eating two servings to five or more a day improved their immune response to the pneumonia vaccine.
- Exercise your arm and shoulder for 15 minutes right before getting the shot. This strengthened people's response to the pneumonia vaccine.
- Get treated for depression if you need help. People with untreated depression had a weaker immune response to the shingles vaccine, compared to those under treatment for their depression.

Flip the switch on allergies

Allergy misery: an immune system mix-up

The trees and ragweed aren't out to get you — your immune system is. You can lay the blame for hay fever, hives, allergic rashes, food allergies, and asthma directly at the feet of your immune cells.

These allergies all strike when your immune system mistakes a harmless substance, like a speck of pollen or a food's protein, for a foreign invader. The first time one of these allergens enters your body, your immune B cells leap into action. They begin churning out antibodies custom made to fit that allergen.

The antibodies attach to mast cells in your skin, respiratory tract, and digestive tract, waiting for the same allergen to invade again. The next time it does, the antibodies latch onto it, triggering the mast cell to release histamine and inflammatory compounds that cause your allergy symptoms.

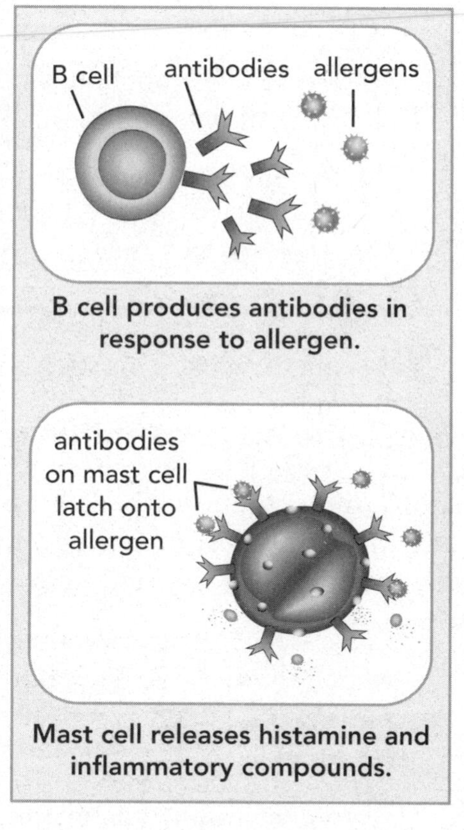

B cell produces antibodies in response to allergen.

Mast cell releases histamine and inflammatory compounds.

Allergies tend to run in families, and they can affect many different parts of your body. Allergic rhinitis, or hay fever, irritates your nose, eyes, mouth, and throat. Food allergies can aggravate your skin, nose, eyes, esophagus, and even your digestive system. Contact dermatitis impacts your skin.

Pollen, dust, animal dander, foods like peanuts and shellfish, mold, medications, and latex cause the most problems. Some of the allergies you have as a child may go away, only to be replaced by new ones as an adult. Thankfully, medicines and simple avoidance techniques can ease your suffering and, in some cases, save your life.

Pain-free solution to seasonal shots

The Food and Drug Administration recently approved a new form of immunotherapy — tablets that dissolve under your tongue. You can now get tablets for ragweed and certain grass allergies. You must take the first dose in your doctor's office in case you have an allergic reaction to it, but you can take the rest at home. The treatment begins three months before allergy season.

Break the cycle of sniffling and sneezing

Stop hiding out during pollen season or struggling year-round with mold and dust mite allergies. It's time to fight back against sneezing, runny noses, and itchy, watery eyes.

- Pin seasonal allergies on pollen. Pollen season generally runs March through October, but trees in the South can begin putting out pollen as early as January. Ragweed is the top fall offender.
- Blame year-round allergies on indoor aggravators, including dust mites, mold, pet dander, dried skin flakes, and roaches.

A runny nose may be the least of your worries if you don't get your allergies under control. Long-lasting congestion can lead to sinus and ear infections, and out-of-control allergies are more likely to develop into asthma.

Treating your allergies could even ease migraines. Migraine sufferers have more frequent and more severe headaches during hay fever season. People who received allergy shots in one study had half as many migraines as those who didn't get shots. So what are you waiting for? Score relief with this winning game plan.

Manage symptoms with meds. Get a jump on your allergies by starting antihistamines and steroid nasal sprays before your symptoms strike. "Allergy sufferers should start taking medication that has worked well for them in the past at least two weeks before the season starts," advises allergist Myron Zitt, past president of the American College of Allergy, Asthma, and Immunology. This gives the drugs time to build up in your bloodstream, making them much more effective once pollen season hits. Stop the medicines between allergy seasons.

- Take short-acting antihistamines 30 minutes before stepping outside, or take long-acting, time-released antihistamines on a regular schedule, rather than as-needed.
- Consider a nasal steroid spray such as Flonase, Nasalcort, or Nasarel if antihistamines alone don't dampen your symptoms. Steroid sprays can boost blood sugar levels, so monitor yours carefully if you have diabetes.
- Take a decongestant pill to ease congestion and reduce swelling in your nose. But keep this in mind — elderly adults sometimes react badly to decongestants. Also avoid them if you have high blood pressure, an enlarged prostate, severe coronary artery disease, or take monoamine oxidase inhibitors (Marplan, Nardil, Emsam, Parnate) for depression.

- Don't use a decongestant nasal spray for hay fever symptoms. It can actually worsen your congestion if taken for more than three days. Stick with decongestant pills.

Talk to an allergist about immunotherapy if the usual medicines can't control your allergies. Allergy shots and other types of immunotherapy desensitize your immune system to specific allergens, so your body stops reacting to them. It's the only treatment that truly cures allergies.

Get a little exercise. Moderate exercise actually dampens your immune reaction to allergens like pollen. Research shows that jogging on a treadmill for 30 minutes triggers your body to release compounds that calm your immune system. Strenuous activity can aggravate asthma and breathing problems.

Take time to relax. Your allergies may flare up when your stress levels spike. "Stress can cause several negative effects on the body, including more symptoms for allergy sufferers," according to Amber Patterson, Assistant Professor of Pediatrics at Ohio State University's College of Medicine. Allergy sufferers in one study saw their symptoms worsen a few days after their stress levels rose.

Try an herb. Butterbur supplements may work as well as over-the-counter antihistamines. In one study, taking a butterbur extract named Ze 339 three times a day — totaling 8 milligrams of the compound petasin — relieved hay fever symptoms as well as Allegra. Only buy supplements that have been processed to remove the toxic pyrrolizidine alkaloids naturally found in this herb.

Wash away allergens. Rinsing your nasal and sinus passages with salt water can help manage your symptoms. Dissolve 1 teaspoon of Kosher or sea salt along with a pinch of baking soda into 2 cups of warm water, either distilled or boiled for three minutes and allowed to cool. Only do this during allergy flare-ups. Rinsing daily for more than a year may actually make you more prone to sinus infections, possibly by washing away too much protective mucus. So can using tap and filtered water. Learn how to prep your rinse water in *Dodge hidden danger in sinus rinse* in the *Get smart about fighting germs* chapter.

Avoid what aggravates you. One of the best ways to conquer your allergies is to avoid what aggravates them. Try these strategies to cut back on sniffling and sneezing.

- Bathe before bed to wash pollen out of your hair and off your skin so it doesn't get on your pillowcase and sheets.
- Invest in HVAC filters with a MERV rating of 11 or 12. These catch dust, pollen, and dander better than lower-rated filters. Change them every three months.
- Control dust mites with a vacuum cleaner that uses a HEPA air filter, and wash sheets and pillowcases weekly in hot water.
- Limit mold by removing houseplants and dried flowers from your bedroom and living areas. Use incandescent light bulbs, not low-wattage CFL or LED bulbs, in closets to help evaporate moisture and prevent mold growth.

Honey — no sweet relief for hay fever

It's an old wives tale that unfortunately isn't true. Eating raw, local honey probably won't improve your allergies. The idea makes sense — desensitizing your immune system to local pollen by exposing it to the small amounts in raw, unprocessed honey. That's how allergy shots work, too.

In this case, theory doesn't translate into reality. The pollen that bees collect is not the kind that aggravates your allergies. That comes from grass, trees, and weeds, which are not pollinated by bees. Tiny amounts of allergy-causing pollen may end up in raw honey by accident, but not enough to desensitize your immune system. In fact, raw honey may cause allergic reactions in some people, perhaps due to pollen or bee parts that wind up in it unintentionally.

Secrets to sneeze-free gardening

Don't let pollen and mold keep you from your favorite hobby. Give your green thumb a workout by putting in plants that won't aggravate your allergies.

Flowers and trees pollinated by bees and other insects are safe bets. They produce large grains of pollen that are easy for bugs, but not wind, to carry. As a result, you aren't likely to inhale them. Weeds, trees, and grasses that rely on wind pollination are the problem. They produce small, lightweight pollen particles that lift easily into the air and head straight for your nose.

Go for bold colors. Plant flowers and shrubs with bright, colorful blooms, such as azalea, hibiscus, zinnia, tulip, sunflower, rose, lilac, daffodil, begonia, geranium, petunia, pansy, salvia, and cactus.

Grow the right grass. Most grasses don't cause allergies, but a few do, including Bermuda, Kentucky bluegrass, Johnson grass, orchard grass, sweet vernal grass, Timothy grass, fescue, and ryegrass. Is your lawn already covered in Kentucky bluegrass? Then stay indoors from late spring to early summer when most grasses release their pollen.

Choose trees carefully. A few trees cause most of the misery from late winter to early summer. Oak, elm, birch, maple, walnut, juniper, cedar, cypress, sycamore, hickory, alder, beech, chestnut, box elder, and sequoia are some of the worst offenders.

Fill your yard instead with crape myrtle, dogwood, fig, fir, pear, apple, magnolia, redbud, palm, and redwood trees. You can also plant the female cultivars of maple, willow, poplar, cottonwood, ash, and box elder. They won't produce the same sneeze-inducing pollen as the males.

Wage war on weeds. Ragweed, especially the low-growing, tooth-leaved kind, is the main cause of fall allergies, but it can't take all the credit. Plaintain, pigweed, lambs-quarters, sagebrush, sheep sorrel, mugwort, and cocklebur also take top allergy honors.

Try to remove as many of these from your landscape as possible, or at least keep them mowed low to lop off the flowers.

Is your sofa making you itch?

That rash on your bottom? Blame it on the leather recliner you just bought. Leather furniture and shoes made in China have been causing allergic rashes around the world. These goods get shipped across thousands of miles of ocean. To inhibit mold growth along the way, Chinese manufacturers sometimes pack leather items with dimethyl fumarate (DMF), much like the silica packets that come in pill bottles. Except some people are allergic to DMF. It leaches into the leather, and from there into your clothes.

Allergic rashes like these are another instance of your immune system protecting you from substances that aren't really a threat. Your skin is home to many specialized immune cells. When your skin touches a substance you're allergic to, even if it's completely harmless, these cells leap into action and attack it, producing the red, itchy rash known as contact dermatitis. You may not get a rash the first or even second time an allergen touches your skin. It may take a while for your immune system to become overly sensitive to the substance.

There's little you can do about itch-inducing leather furniture except toss it to the curb, since DMF can take years to evaporate. Fortunately, that's not the case with most other allergens. Here's how to guard against the worst of them.

Hidden nickel. Stephen Katz, director of the National Institute of Arthritis and Musculoskeletal and Skin Diseases, says nickel is the most common cause of contact dermatitis. "Why? Because of ear piercing." Many cheap earrings contain nickel. Your immune system can become sensitive to it over time. Once you are allergic, you'll also react to the nickel in zippers, buttons, chrome-plated items, kitchen utensils, mobile phones, tablet computers, and 14 karat and 18 karat gold.

Buy earrings with surgical steel posts to avoid this problem. If you already have a nickel allergy, coat earring posts, metal buttons, and metal snaps with clear nail polish to create a barrier between them and your skin.

Everyday fragrances. They're not just in perfume. Food, makeup, lotion, soap, insecticide, antiseptics, and even dental products can all contain rash-causing fragrances. One of the most common, linalool, is in up to 80 percent of household cleaners and hygiene products, like soaps, shampoos, and conditioners. And one in 20 people may be allergic to it.

"Some people can shower with shower cream that contains linalool and never develop an allergy, but we know that the risk increases as the exposure to the substance increases," explains dermatologist Johanna Bråred Christensson. Linalool is most likely to bother you if it has been stored for a long time or exposed to air. "Avoid buying large packs of soap and shower cream, and always replace the top after using a bottle," suggests Christensson.

As for other fragrances, don't count on products labeled "hypoallergenic" or "unscented." They may still contain small amounts of scent. Check the ingredient list for Balsam of Peru and other fragrances. And rinse thoroughly when you bathe or wash your hands.

Pesky preservatives. Hygienic wet wipes are more popular than ever, but they're causing more rashes, too. The culprit is the chemical preservative methylisothiazolinone (MI), also found in liquid soap, hair products, sunscreen, cosmetics, cleaners, and laundry products. "In the last two or three years, we've suddenly seen a big increase in people with this type of allergy," says Matthew Zirwas, of Ohio State University's Wexner Medical Center. Suspect MI if you develop a poison ivy-like rash on your fingers, hands, face, buttocks, or genitals. Stop using moist wipes for one month and see if your rash improves.

Mild rashes usually go away on their own, but see a doctor if it occurs on your face, lingers for several days, is very uncomfortable, looks infected, or develops shortly after you start taking a new medicine. In the meantime, try these simple, at-home treatments to soothe contact dermatitis.

- Apply calamine lotion or an anti-itch cream with at least 1 percent hydrocortisone.
- Take an oral antihistamine, such as Benadryl, if topical creams don't stop the itching.
- Dip a soft, white cloth in a mixture of cool water and 2 tablespoons of baking soda. Wring it out and apply to the rash.
- Soak in a cool, not cold, bath with baking soda or colloidal oatmeal.
- Try to avoid scratching the rash. Trim your nails to keep from breaking the skin or cover the rash with gauze and bandages.
- Wear smooth, cotton clothing to avoid irritating your skin further.

High-tech help to ward off rashes

Use your computer or mobile phone to steer clear of allergy-causing chemicals in everyday products. The Contact Allergen Replacement Database (CARD) tracks the ingredients in nearly 5,500 skin care products. You can use it to search for products that are free of the fragrances, preservatives, and other substances you're allergic to.

Access CARD through your computer's Web browser at *http://card.preventice.com*, or download the app to your iPhone, iPod Touch, or iPad. You can access the database for free the first year and for a small monthly fee after.

4 tips for faster asthma relief

You have more control over asthma than you think. From foods that soothe inflamed airways to simple tips on taking your medicine, you have tools at your fingertips to help you live a normal life.

Some people have allergic asthma, where an allergen such as pollen, pet dander, mold, or dust mites triggers an attack. Their immune systems spot the allergen and think it's an invading germ. Immune cells attack, releasing histamine and other chemicals that make airways narrow and inflamed.

Others have nonallergic asthma, where an irritant like exercise, stress, or cold air sets off an attack. In this case, your airways twitch when they come in contact with the irritant. This twitching makes the muscles around your airways contract, putting the squeeze on breathing.

No matter what causes your attacks, the result is the same — coughing, shortness of breath, chest tightness, and wheezing. The dangers of asthma come not just from attacks but also from long-term lung damage. The longer your airways remain inflamed, the thicker and narrower they get, and the less they are able to relax.

Experts say prevention is the best strategy. Avoid what you know aggravates your asthma, and see an allergist if your attacks are severe, unpredictable, or occurring more than twice a week. These tips can help you manage your symptoms.

Trim the fat. People with severe, persistent asthma eat about the same number of calories as healthy people, but they eat much more fat and sodium and much less fiber and potassium. Research links this unhealthy combination with worse lung function and more inflammation in the airways. Diets high in fat, salt, and sugar make your body produce more inflammatory compounds — bad news for asthma sufferers. On the other hand, diets rich in fish and fiber may improve asthma and lung function.

And consider this — not all fats are bad. Foods full of alpha-tocopherol, a type of vitamin E, can actually calm inflammation in your lungs. Learn more about it in *Breathe easy with this 'E'ssential vitamin* in the *Vitamin-rich foods: what you should be eating now* chapter.

Fight against gasping. Resisting the urge to take deep, gasping breaths during an attack can ease symptoms and lead to healthier lungs. "Deep, rapid breathing causes a drop in carbon dioxide gas in the blood. That makes a person feel dizzy and short of breath," explains Thomas Ritz, clinical psychologist at Southern Methodist University.

Ritz and his colleagues used biofeedback to teach people with asthma to take shallow, short breaths during an attack. It worked. "Patients in our study increased their carbon dioxide and reduced their symptoms," he says. Over six months, they experienced healthy changes in their lung tissue, too. Shallow breathing techniques could even reduce your need for a rescue inhaler. It's not easy to override the instinct to gasp during an attack, so you may need the help of biofeedback training. Ask your doctor for details.

Make taking your meds a morning ritual. Remembering to use your steroid inhaler daily is crucial for controlling the long-term lung inflammation caused by asthma. But only one in three people over age 60 remembers to use it. Scientists asked those successful seniors how they remembered their medicine so faithfully, and they uncovered a few good tips.

- take your inhaled steroids at the same time every day.
- take it along with your other medications.
- make it part of your morning routine, when you brush your teeth or eat breakfast, for instance.
- keep your inhaler in a specific place, like your bathroom.

Drink ginger tea. Compounds in ginger may make your asthma medication more effective by relaxing the muscles in your airways. Ginger compounds block an enzyme that keeps your airways inflamed and prevents them from relaxing. Ginger may not be strong enough on its own to end an asthma attack, but experts think it could make beta-agonist drugs more effective at easing symptoms.

Foods that affect your seasonal allergies

One in three people with seasonal allergies also have oral allergy syndrome. Their immune systems confuse the proteins in certain foods with the proteins in pollen, triggering an attack. You could be one of them if you develop sniffles, sneezes, or an itchy mouth, lips, or throat after eating certain raw or fresh fruits and other foods.

People allergic to	May react to
tree pollen	cherries, apricots, kiwis, oranges, plums, hazelnuts, and walnuts
oak or birch pollen	carrots, celery, almonds, apples, peaches, and pears
grass pollen	melons, tomatoes, and oranges
ragweed	bananas, cantaloupe, cucumber, zucchini, and chamomile tea

Most reactions are minor and harmless, says allergist Joseph Leija. But if you develop trouble breathing or an itchy rash, "go to a board-certified allergist or, in extreme cases, straight to the emergency room."

Tiny insect triggers deadly allergy

A tick bite could suddenly make you allergic to red meat. It's an odd but increasingly common food allergy. Some lone star ticks carry a sugar called alpha-gal in their guts. When they bite, that sugar crosses into your bloodstream, where your immune system sees it and tags it as an invader. The next time alpha-gal enters your body, your immune system mounts an all-out attack.

Unfortunately, red meats such as beef, pork, lamb, and venison naturally contain alpha-gal. Once you are allergic, eating these meats can trigger something as mild as a stuffy nose, sneezing, stomach cramps, or hives, or as serious as anaphylaxis — vomiting, diarrhea, trouble breathing, and a dangerous drop in blood pressure. The reaction may not start until four to six hours after your meal. Poultry is safe to eat, although some people react to milk, even in small amounts.

Red meat isn't the only food allergy that might surprise you. Beware these little-known allergens.

- Lupin. This legume is closely related to peanuts and soybeans, and it's commonly used in gluten-free foods in place of flour. People allergic to peanuts may also react to lupin. Check ingredient lists for lupin or lupine.
- Pesticides on fruits and vegetables. Pesticides that contain antibiotics can pose a problem if you're allergic to drugs like penicillin. Wash your food thoroughly before eating it, and consider buying organic.

Get to a doctor or emergency clinic immediately if you have an allergic reaction to food. Then follow up with an allergist. Carry an EpiPen with you at all times.

As for red meat allergies, avoid tick-prone areas and activities. Repeated tick bites can make you even more allergic to alpha-gal.

Autoimmune diseases: how to survive and thrive

What to do when your body turns on you

Most people's immune systems hum along without a hitch. But 23.5 million Americans aren't so lucky. Their immune cells turn against them, attacking organs, joints, and other tissue. The result — one of more than 80 autoimmune disorders.

Normally, your immune system destroys immune cells that go rogue and attack healthy tissue, but a few always slip through the cracks. Experts think a combination of genetics, environment, and lifestyle triggers these broken cells to begin attacking the body.

- Some people's genes make them more susceptible to immune system malfunctions. That helps explain why some autoimmune diseases run in families.
- Those faulty genes then react with something in your environment, say a chemical or virus, that sets off your immune system. Estrogen may play a role, too, since women are more likely to develop autoimmune diseases than men.
- Your lifestyle has an impact, as well. For example, being extremely overweight makes your immune system more likely to attack healthy cells. Obesity also generates inflammation that can worsen autoimmune diseases or hinder their treatment.

Once these elements collide, they trigger a cascade of events that ends with your body trying to destroy itself. Autoimmune illnesses can target specific organs or affect your entire body.

type 1 diabetes	pancreas
multiple sclerosis	brain and spinal cord
psoriasis	skin
lupus	tissues throughout the body, including joints, skin, kidneys, heart, and lungs
Hashimoto and Graves' diseases	thyroid
inflammatory bowel disease	digestive tract
rheumatoid arthritis	joints throughout the body

Each disease is different, but many share core symptoms of fatigue, dizziness, and low-grade fever. Three can cause hair loss that has nothing to do with aging, including lupus, alopecia areata, and Hashimoto disease, all of which are treatable. Autoimmune diseases have no simple solutions, but experts know how you can better manage your symptoms.

Rest up. First, get plenty of sleep each night. Most people need seven to nine hours. Don't short yourself. Your body uses this downtime to repair its tissues and joints. Being well-rested also lowers your stress levels, which can ease symptoms, and helps your body better fight off other illnesses. Learn how to build good sleep habits by reading *Take these smart steps to sounder sleep* in the *Sleep right to save your life* chapter.

Stress less. Stress and anxiety can cause symptoms to flare up in some autoimmune diseases. Do what you can to eliminate stress in your life, and consider joining a support group for people with your condition. Sharing strategies and concerns with people who understand may help lower your anxiety levels.

Rheumatoid arthritis: tips for living better

You thought you had the flu, and now you've developed swollen, achy joints. These are classic signs of an autoimmune disease known as rheumatoid arthritis (RA). If you have these symptoms, be sure your doctor checks for RA. It's more crippling than osteoarthritis, and the right diagnosis will mean the right treatment.

It starts when your immune cells attack the synovial membrane surrounding your joints. During the battle, these cells release the same toxins they use to kill bacteria and viruses. That can cause flu-like symptoms — weakness, low-grade fever, fatigue, and loss of appetite. Before long, you'll begin to feel the disease in your joints in the form of heat, swelling, pain, and redness.

Chronic joint inflammation makes the synovial membrane thicken. All the while, your immune cells keep releasing toxins. This combination gradually deforms your joints by breaking down the cartilage, tendons, ligaments, and even bone. Eventually, the inflammation can spread to your tear ducts, salivary glands, or the lining of your chest.

A more common form of arthritis, known as osteoarthritis, usually hits large, weight-bearing joints. RA, on the other hand, tends to strike small joints, such as toes, wrists, and knuckles. And it affects the same joint on both sides of your body. If you develop RA in your right hand, you'll probably get it in your left.

Experts have yet to pinpoint only one cause. Like other autoimmune diseases, it's triggered by a combination of genes, environment, and lifestyle. Certain genes make you more likely to develop this disease. If yours do, a bacterial or viral infection may set off an immune malfunction that leads to RA. Unhealthy habits, like smoking and eating too much red meat, make your immune system more likely to go haywire and attack your joints. And, for some reason, women are much more likely to get it than men.

You can't do anything about your genes or your gender, but you can change your lifestyle in ways that will lower your RA risk.

- Avoid sugary sodas. Out of more than 186,000 women, those who drank one or more sugary sodas a day were more likely to develop RA, particularly after age 55. Diet sodas had no effect.
- Quit smoking, the sooner the better. Even light smoking raises your risk. Women who smoked seven or fewer cigarettes a day were more than twice as likely to get RA. Women who had quit smoking at least 15 years earlier cut that risk by 30 percent.
- Get down to a healthy weight. Obesity is a major risk factor for rheumatoid arthritis, especially in women. Fat cells churn out compounds that impact inflammation and your immune system.

Family doctors don't see many cases of rheumatoid arthritis. So if you suspect you have it, get a referral to a rheumatologist right away. They can diagnose and start you on medications to prevent joint damage. While there, ask your specialist if these promising treatments could ease your pain or slow the disease.

Find relief with fish oil. Taking high doses of fish oil alongside your regular RA medicines could make the disease more likely to enter remission. EPA and DHA, the omega-3 fatty acids in fish oil, squash inflammatory compounds in your body.

In one study, people with newly diagnosed rheumatoid arthritis took 10 milliliters of fish oil daily with their regular RA drugs for one year. They were twice as likely to enter remission and less likely to have their RA drugs stop working compared to people not taking fish oil. That's important, because when your body stops responding to first-line RA drugs, you could wind up needing very expensive biological drugs. Fish oil could help cheaper, front-line medicines remain effective for longer.

On average, people in this study took a total of 3.7 grams (g) of EPA and DHA a day. High doses of fish oil may thin your blood and increase your risk of stroke, so talk to your doctor before trying it.

Chase away pain with GLA. Your body uses essential fatty acids such as gamma linolenic acid (GLA) to make compounds that control inflammation and pain. Some fatty acids increase pain and inflammation while others — like GLA — decrease it. Several studies suggest that GLA supplements improve RA symptoms, especially when taken with your regular arthritis medicines.

People in most studies took 2 to 3 g of GLA daily. Experts suggest splitting this into several doses throughout the day, and taking each dose with food. This supplement may thin your blood, so ask your rheumatologist if it's safe for you. If so, look for purified GLA supplements. Borage and evening primrose oils also contain GLA but not in large enough amounts to treat RA.

Double-down on vitamin D. Want to get more pain relief than drugs alone can offer? Consider adding 500 international units (IU) of vitamin D3 to your daily regimen of RA medicines. In one study, people who did experienced greater pain relief after three months than those taking drugs alone.

Most immune cells have receptors specifically made for locking onto vitamin D. This nutrient makes your immune cells more tolerant of healthy tissue and less likely to attack it in an autoimmune reaction. Vitamin D also boosts your immune response to real invaders, like infectious bacteria.

Roughly 65 percent of people with RA are vitamin D deficient. Low levels may speed up the destruction of cartilage and bone in joints with RA. Get your vitamin D level tested, and ask your doctor about taking supplements if you're deficient.

Stay active when you're able. Moderate exercise during times of remission strengthens your bones and helps protect against osteoporosis, a serious danger if you take steroids for your RA. Water aerobics are perfect because the water takes some of the load off your joints.

Of course, you can't work out during flare ups. Instead, try bending and straightening your joints. Gentle stretches, such as opening and closing your hands, keep your joints flexible and help maintain your range of motion.

Don't be fooled by arthritis 'cures'

Pharmacies sell copper bracelets and magnetic wrist bands, so they must work, right? Sadly, no. A gold-standard study has shown once and for all that these devices don't help rheumatoid arthritis (RA) symptoms. Seventy people with RA took turns wearing an ordinary wrist band, a magnetic one, or a copper bracelet for five weeks each. None of them improved joint pain, physical function, or inflammation levels.

So why do people swear by them? Two reasons — hope and timing. The placebo effect is powerful. Simply believing that something works can make you feel better.

Second, autoimmune diseases like rheumatoid arthritis naturally go through periods where symptoms worsen then improve on their own. "People normally begin wearing [these devices] during a flare-up period. As their symptoms subside naturally over time, they confuse this with a therapeutic effect," explains Stewart Richmond, a researcher at the University of York in Great Britain who headed the study.

5 proven ways to take control of lupus

Overwhelming fatigue, painful joints, and a rash that looks like a bad sunburn all make lupus hard to live with, but you don't have to suffer in silence. A few simple changes in your habits and your diet will help put you back in the driver's seat.

In lupus, your immune system attacks organs and tissues throughout your body. There are two main types. Systemic lupus erythematosus (SLE) affects many areas, such as your joints, kidneys, hair, and skin. The attack causes widespread symptoms, ranging from painful, swollen joints and fever to a rash and fatigue. Cutaneous lupus solely affects your skin, causing rashes, lesions, hair loss, and sensitivity to light.

An astounding nine out of 10 people with lupus are women. Most develop it during their childbearing years, between the ages of 15 and 45, whereas men tend to get it either in childhood or after age 50. It's also more common in African-American, Latina, Asian, and Native American women.

Some people are genetically more likely to get lupus, but your environment has a lot to do with whether that happens. Smoking, stress, viruses, and sunlight can all trigger the disease in people prone to it. Long-term use of pesticides around your home and workplace raise your risk, too, even if you aren't the one spraying them.

Some of the same things linked to the development of lupus can also trigger painful flares — working too hard, resting too little, stress, exposure to ultraviolet rays, and fighting off an infection or injury.

Doctors treat lupus with anti-inflammatory drugs, immune-suppressing medications, and corticosteroids, like prednisone. But you can do plenty on your own to tamp down flares and keep your disease in remission.

Stop smoking. This will have a bigger impact on lupus than any other change you make. Here are five ways smoking affects your health:

- raises your risk of infections, including pneumonia and bronchitis
- increases your chance of heart problems, such as heart attack and coronary artery disease
- narrows your blood vessels and worsens circulation, both problems for people with lupus

- makes you more likely to have a stroke
- raises your blood pressure, which puts more strain on lupus-damaged kidneys

People with lupus already have higher risks of all of these conditions — stroke, infections, heart problems, high blood pressure, and many more. Why stack the deck against yourself further? Quit smoking, and you'll see immediate benefits.

Increase your vitamin D. People with lupus often have to avoid sunlight, which can leave them deficient in this major nutrient. Experts suggest taking a calcium-plus-vitamin D supplement to prevent bone loss if you treat your lupus long-term with steroids. Getting more vitamin D may also quiet lupus activity and inflammation. Ask your doctor to test your blood levels and recommend a supplement, if necessary.

Savor some citrus. Load up on vitamin C-rich foods like oranges and kiwis when your lupus is in remission. In a study that included 241 women with lupus, those who got the most vitamin C from food were the least likely to experience a flare. Vitamin C supplements didn't offer the same protection.

Indulge in yogurt. Eating foods that contain the bacteria *Lactobacillus* could reduce flares and improve lupus symptoms. Research shows that mice with a lupus-like disease have fewer *Lactobacillus* and more *Clostridia* bacteria in their guts than healthy mice. That imbalance is worse in the beginning and end stages of lupus. This doesn't prove that gut bacteria trigger the disease, but it does suggest that eating foods like yogurt that contain live *Lactobacillus* cultures may soothe symptoms.

Guard against lights. You know sunlight can trigger a lupus flare. But did you know halogen bulbs, fluorescent tube lights, and even energy-saving compact fluorescent bulbs (CFLs) can aggravate lupus?

They all emit ultraviolet (UV) radiation, which damages the DNA in skin cells. This DNA damage sets off a false alarm in the immune system of people with lupus. Immune cells attack in response to the "threat," causing inflammation, redness, and lesions similar to a bad sunburn.

Take steps to protect yourself.

- When outdoors, wear sunscreen with an SPF of 30 or higher that protects against both ultraviolet A (UVA) and ultraviolet B (UVB) rays.
- Avoid direct sunlight on your skin between 10 a.m. and 4 p.m.
- Wear broad-brimmed hats in stores and office buildings with fluorescent lights.
- Put acrylic, not glass, covers over fluorescent bulbs and tube lights at home to block their UV rays. Glass covers won't block the radiation.

Drug-induced lupus: a case of mistaken identity

Worried you might have lupus? Take a look in your medicine cabinet. Certain medications can cause drug-induced lupus if taken continuously for months or years. These include:

- hydralazine (Apresoline) for high blood pressure.
- quinidine (Quiniglute) and procainamide (Pronestyl, Procanbid) for irregular heartbeat.
- phenytoin (Dilantin) for seizures.
- etanercept (Enbrel) and adalimumab (Humira) for psoriasis and rheumatoid arthritis.

Unlike regular lupus, drug-induced symptoms generally go away within a few weeks of stopping the medicine causing the problem. Never stop taking a prescription drug on your own. Instead, ask your doctor to switch you to a different medication.

Drug-free tips to ease psoriasis itch

Psoriasis doesn't discriminate. This autoimmune disease doesn't care if you're rich or poor, famous or unknown. Just ask top golfer Phil Mickelson. He was diagnosed with psoriatic arthritis one week after a major tournament. The right treatments helped him keep playing — and winning.

In psoriasis, your immune cells mistake your skin cells for germs and attack them. Your skin churns out an excess of skin cells in response. This most often occurs on hands and feet but can happen anywhere on your body, including your scalp. It's more than just a skin disease. Up to 30 percent of people with psoriasis also develop psoriatic arthritis in their joints. Psoriasis raises your risk of diabetes, heart attack, liver disease, kidney disease, vascular problems, and chronic obstructive pulmonary disease (COPD), as well. The larger the affected area of skin, the higher your risk of these other illnesses.

Unfortunately, there's no cure. Psoriasis lasts a lifetime, flaring up during periods of illness or stress then dying down again. That doesn't mean you can't control the course of the disease. These simple tips will help you tackle the dry, itchy skin of psoriasis — and none of them involves spending money on expensive creams.

Soak up some sun. Julie Moore, a dermatologist at Gottlieb Memorial Hospital, has some simple advice. "The sun is one of the best treatments for psoriasis, so in summer I encourage my patients to sit out on the deck and give their affected areas a good sun bath." It doesn't take much. "Twenty to 30 minutes is adequate to improve the skin; you do not need to sit out for hours."

Get cozy with gut bugs. Probiotics containing the bacterium *Bifidobacterium infantis* may help control psoriasis. These beneficial bugs may influence your body to make more regulatory T cells, special immune cells that reign in out-of-control immune reactions. Look for probiotic supplements like Align that specifically contain this bug.

Stamp out stress. The nerve endings in your skin release chemicals that control the immune cells living in your skin. Stress makes these nerve endings release more chemicals, and that, in turn, causes skin inflammation. Stress is one sure way to worsen your psoriasis. Gentle relaxation exercises like yoga or tai chi may help.

Drop the salt shaker. Salt may cause your body to make more inflammatory immune cells, worsening autoimmune diseases like psoriasis. In mice, eating a high-salt diet speeds up the development of an autoimmune disease similar to multiple sclerosis, according to a recent Yale School of Medicine study. More research is needed to connect all the dots, but cutting back on salt is generally safe and healthy.

Slim down. Gaining weight makes psoriasis more severe, whereas losing weight can relieve symptoms and reduce the amount of skin affected by the disease. Whittling down to a healthy weight also slashes your risk of heart problems and heart-related death, which is higher in people with severe psoriasis. Learn how to shed pounds safely in *Step 3: Lose the fat*.

Can immune cells cause Parkinson's?

Intriguing new research suggests Parkinson's disease (PD) may be partly autoimmune. People with Parkinson's have less dopamine in their brains, a chemical necessary to control movement and coordination. They also have fewer brain cells that make dopamine, compared to people without PD.

Some scientists now think the immune system may mistakenly target and kill the brain cells that make dopamine. This doesn't explain the entire disease, but it may be an important clue in one day unraveling it.

Reign in runaway blood sugar

People with type 1 diabetes are living longer than ever — if they work to keep their blood sugar under control. Unlike type 2 diabetes, which is brought on by lifestyle choices, type 1 occurs when your immune system destroys the beta cells in your pancreas that make insulin.

Sugar, or glucose, is the main fuel for cells. Insulin moves sugar from your bloodstream into each cell. Without insulin, you can't survive. People with type 1 diabetes need daily insulin injections to provide what their bodies can no longer make.

Type 1 accounts for only 5 to 10 percent of diabetes cases. Your genes may make you more likely to get it, especially if your father or grandfather had it. But DNA alone doesn't cause it. Experts think a childhood virus may change your immune system. When you catch the same virus later on, it could trigger your immune cells to attack your pancreas.

Stay on top of important numbers. Controlling your blood sugar is key to living a long life with diabetes. Experts generally recommend keeping your hemoglobin A1c level below 7 percent and your fasting blood sugar between 90 and 130 milligrams (mg) per deciliter (dL). The American Geriatrics Society says people over age 65 can aim for an A1c level between 7 and 7.5 percent. In most cases, the closer you can get to those goals, the better. People with type 1 diabetes who kept their blood sugar tightly controlled:

- were less likely to develop problems with their vision, kidneys, nerves, and circulation.
- slashed their risk of stroke, nonfatal heart attack, and fatal heart disease by more than half.
- suffered less mental decline with age.

Going too low can be dangerous, especially for older adults. Ask your doctor what your targets should be. Hypoglycemic (low blood sugar) episodes raise your risk of dementia, possibly by starving your brain of nutrients. Repeated bouts of hypoglycemia dull your body's response to these drops, making you less likely to notice when your blood sugar gets dangerously low. Your doctor may recommend raising your blood sugar targets if you have had several recent bouts of hypoglycemia.

Consider getting a continuous glucose monitor. It may do more to lower your A1c levels than the finger-stick method of testing. The monitors feature an alarm that warns you when your blood sugar drops too low or shoots too high.

Get up and get moving. Exercise can shave another 0.6 percent off your A1c level, plus lower your blood pressure, cholesterol, and triglycerides. Talk to your doctor before beginning an exercise routine to make sure it's safe for you. If you have:

- diabetic retinopathy, avoid vigorous aerobic or resistance exercises and use only light weights.
- nerve damage in your arms or legs (peripheral neuropathy), try walking at a moderate speed. Walking should not harm your feet, as long as you don't have foot sores or injuries. Wear good shoes and check your feet daily for sores.
- autonomic neuropathy, have your heart checked before you crank up the intensity on your regular workouts.

Check your blood sugar before each exercise session. If it's below 100 mg/dL, eat a small, carbohydrate-based snack like graham crackers or fruit before exercising. Physical activity can drop your blood sugar even lower, then lead to a sharp spike afterward. Eating a pre-workout snack helps avoid this roller coaster.

Can sunshine vitamin block MS?

The autoimmune disease multiple sclerosis (MS) is most common in countries that lie farthest from the equator — and now experts think they know why. Your body makes vitamin D from sunshine, and the amount of vitamin D in your blood impacts the development and severity of MS. Countries far from the equator get less sun.

In MS, your immune system attacks the sheath that surrounds nerve cells and helps them send signals controlling your muscles and speech. Vitamin D seems to prevent these attacking immune cells from traveling to your brain, where they can do the most damage.

Researchers are conducting studies now to learn whether vitamin D supplements can help people with MS. In the meantime, ask your doctor to test your vitamin D levels and prescribe supplements if you need them.

Foods that soothe an angry gut

Your gut houses a huge portion of your immune system. When immune cells go awry in your intestines, they cause Crohn's disease and ulcerative colitis (UC), two conditions collectively known as inflammatory bowel disease (IBD).

Roughly 1.4 million Americans suffer from IBD. Genes play a role, but your environment may matter more. Experts think a virus, bacteria, food allergy, or something else in your surroundings triggers your immune system to attack your digestive tract. Once turned "on," your immune system doesn't turn "off" properly. That leads to chronic inflammation in your intestines. When the attack and inflammation occur in your small intestine, it's called Crohn's disease. When it strikes your large intestine, it's ulcerative colitis.

Both illnesses go through periods of flare ups, marked by abdominal pain and bloody diarrhea, and remission. During flares, immune cells kill the "good" bacteria living in your gut, leaving lots of room for bad ones, such as *E. coli*, to take over. This explosion of *E. coli* may be to blame for the diarrhea that characterizes IBD.

Anti-inflammatory, corticosteroid, antibiotic, and immune-suppressing drugs all help control IBD, but what you eat matters, too. Many people with IBD eat overly strict diets, cutting out foods they don't necessarily need to avoid. Experts suggest that people with Crohn's disease try to avoid:

- foods loaded with animal fat, such as high-fat dairy and meats.
- stringy or fibrous foods packed with insoluble fiber, such as green beans, corn on the cob, potato skins, wheat bran, tomato skins, and orange piths.
- processed, high-fat foods because they usually contain emulsifiers, detergents that can alter the behavior of your gut bacteria.

Dish detergent also contains emulsifiers, so be sure to rinse your dishes and silverware thoroughly before using them.

Different foods tend to cause flare ups in people with ulcerative colitis. If you have it:

- eat red meat and processed meat no more than once a week.
- avoid margarine.
- try cutting out milk and cheese, and see if your symptoms improve.

Along with careful eating, be sure to get plenty of good-quality sleep. Poor sleep disrupts your immune system. That may explain why people with ulcerative colitis who consistently sleep poorly are twice as likely to suffer a flare up within six months.

Step 6: Disease-proof your body

4 changes that can save your life

Lifestyle medicine is the future of chronic disease management.

It sounds trendy, doesn't it? Lifestyle medicine — like it's some kind of treatment-of-the-month. Or perhaps available only to the rich and famous. But this "new" medical discipline is serious stuff meant for every single person on the planet. And it's new only in the sense that the health care system has just recently embraced it.

First, it will help if you understand what chronic diseases are and how they impact health in a global way. The word "chronic" comes from the Greek *chronos*, meaning time. And that is what sets these diseases apart — they are usually slow to progress and can last a long time.

The big three chronic diseases are diabetes, heart disease, and cancer, and together, they are responsible for more than 25 million deaths in the world each year. According to the Centers for Disease Control and Prevention, they are among the most common, costly, and preventable of all health problems in the United States. Here's how the individual conditions break down:

- Diabetes is the seventh leading cause of death in the United States.
- Every year, more people die from heart disease than from any other cause.
- Cancer caused 8.2 million deaths worldwide in 2012, and the World Health Organization expects the number of cancer cases to hit 22 million by the year 2032.

These are sobering statistics. And all the more regrettable because so many of these deaths could be prevented — just by changing four lifestyle behaviors.

- tobacco use
- a lack of exercise
- an unhealthy diet
- excessive alcohol use

These four risk factors are behind all three top chronic diseases. And that's where lifestyle medicine comes in. Dean Ornish, author of *Dr. Dean Ornish's Program for Reversing Heart Disease*, said, "The body has a remarkable ability to heal itself if we simply stop doing what's causing the problem." And in this case, unhealthy behaviors are causing the problem.

Tobacco. While it's common knowledge smoking is related to at least 16 types of cancer, not everyone is aware it's also a risk factor for developing type 2 diabetes. In addition, nearly 20 percent of all deaths from heart disease are related to tobacco use.

Exercise. Stay active, and research shows it will reduce your risk of chronic disease not only by helping control your weight but also by directly impacting hormones.

Four out of five adults don't participate in leisure-time activities that meet the federal Physical Activity Guidelines for Americans — 2.5 hours a week of moderate aerobic activity plus muscle-strengthening exercises at least two days a week.

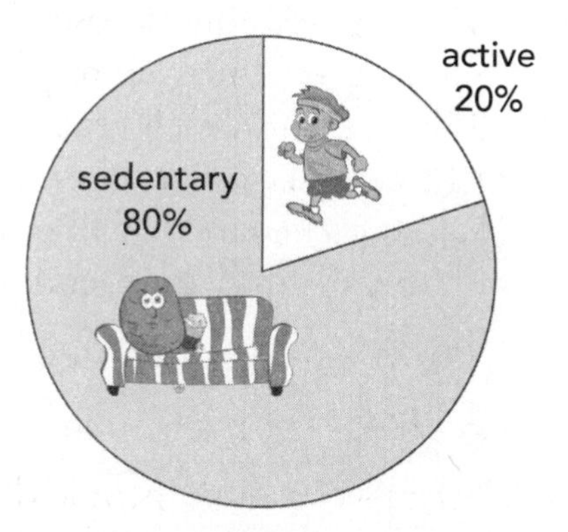

Alcohol. Drinking in moderation can be a positive thing in terms of heart disease risk, inflammation, and insulin resistance. However, too much tips the scales into the danger zone for high blood pressure, diabetes, colon cancer, breast cancer, and mouth and throat cancers.

Diet. Eating whole-grain foods, legumes, vegetables, and fruits while limiting red meat, full-fat dairy, and sugars means you'll maintain a healthier weight and lower your risk of all three of these chronic diseases.

Sixty-eight percent of adults are overweight or obese, which means they have a BMI of 25 or higher.

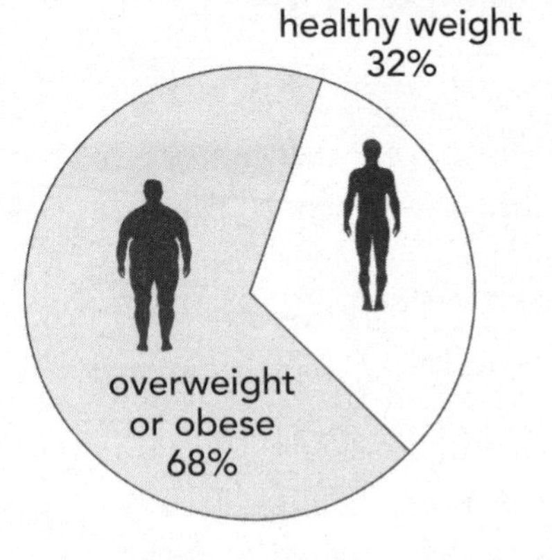

Lifestyle medicine is all about addressing behaviors like these. It doesn't necessarily replace traditional medical treatments, it simply fills the gap left by drugs and clinical practices, encouraging people like you to make choices that will improve your health and quality of life.

Among other things, taking the lifestyle medicine approach means:

- you are an active partner in your care and take on most of the responsibility for your good health.
- your entire lifestyle is examined and adjusted.
- you may be asked to embrace big changes.
- you must commit to changes for the long-term.
- medication may only be a small part of your care.

This concept has become so important that the American Cancer Society, the American Diabetes Association, and the American Heart Association are working together to define a set of clear lifestyle strategies to fight chronic disease. They hope this will help people make better sense of the often confusing and contradictory health messages in the world today.

Inflammation: stamp out the source of disease

Defuse this hidden time bomb

Would it surprise you to learn that a common thread links three of the deadliest diseases facing people today? Experts say chronic inflammation is a shared factor in cancer, heart disease, and diabetes. If you prevent or gain control of this inflammation, you'll not only toughen your overall defenses against these and other diseases, but reduce your risk of dying from them.

You know all about acute inflammation. This is your body's immediate response to some kind of injury, like a cut. Your skin turns red and maybe becomes a little warm and swollen. Or perhaps you catch a cold and start to sniffle and run a temperature. Eventually your amazing immune system does its job. Your wounds mend or the virus is destroyed, and these signs of inflammation fade away. It really is extraordinary, isn't it? With no conscious effort on your part, you are healed.

Chronic inflammation, on the other hand, is practically invisible and can last for months, even years. As it churns away inside your body, the long-term damage can be devastating.

Cancer. Think of sunburn turning into skin cancer, ulcerative colitis changing to colon cancer, acid reflux triggering esophageal cancer, and cigarette smoke causing lung cancer. Many cancers begin with inflammation triggered by an infection or some type of physical or chemical irritant. Cells in the area of inflammation can't live in this new, damaged, and "uncomfortable" environment so they must adapt, a benign process called metaplasia. At this point, the situation is not cancerous. However, in some cases, metaplasia is followed by a much more alarming cell change called dysplasia, which is frequently cancer in its earliest form.

Tests for inflammation confirm this link to cancer. For instance, men with chronic prostate tissue inflammation had almost twice the risk of developing prostate cancer as men without inflammation, one study showed.

Heart disease. Your blood vessels allow life-giving oxygen and nutrients to reach every cell in your body. When they become blocked with cholesterol and other substances from your blood, or damaged by bacterial or viral infection, your immune system leaps into action, sending white blood cells to the rescue. Some experts believe when these cells linger in an area because of persistent inflammation, they set off a series of events that further damage the vessel walls, causing even more plaque to form, and leading to a heart attack or stroke.

Inflammation is so important in heart disease that testing levels of inflammation markers, like C-reactive protein, has become a routine and vital part of medical care.

Diabetes. Certain immune cells, called macrophages, are designed to fight bacteria or viruses. If these macrophages migrate into your fat cells and liver tissue, they can release communication molecules that cause the surrounding cells to become insulin resistant, a first step in developing diabetes. The relationship between inflammation and diabetes was confirmed when scientists found masses of macrophages in the fat cells of people with type 2 diabetes.

In addition to these three major diseases, inflammation is associated with obesity; psychological disorders like depression, schizophrenia, and autism; Alzheimer's disease; asthma; and autoimmune diseases like rheumatoid arthritis and celiac disease.

So what can you do to protect yourself from this potentially deadly chronic inflammation? Diet is key, and you'll read about that later in this chapter. Here are some other inflammation-fighting strategies.

- Talk with your doctor about taking nonsteroidal anti-inflammatory drugs (NSAIDs) like ibuprofen, naproxen, aspirin, or magnesium salicylate. She can monitor the potential long-term side effects.
- Find an aerobic exercise you love and can stick with. Experts believe you need to get moving at least three times a week with each session lasting 30 to 60 minutes. Try brisk walking, cycling, or swimming.
- Start doing resistance training. You don't have to pump iron at the gym, although that works very well. All you really have to do is use your own body weight. Leg lifts, wall push-ups, and working with elastic bands all qualify as strength training and will lower your body's levels of inflammation.
- Combine aerobics and resistance training. It's much more effective than either strategy alone, one study found.
- Quit smoking.
- Find ways to reduce stress, depression, and anxiety. One way is to practice yoga. It reduced inflammation in breast cancer survivors by as much as 20 percent over a 12-week period.
- Get enough quality sleep.
- Take fish oil supplements

6 diet tricks help you beat the heat

Make these easy changes to your diet, and you'll put out the flames of chronic inflammation.

- Stay away from foods high in saturated fat. Specifically, eat less meat. A recent study out of Spain showed the more animal protein in a test diet, the higher the inflammation levels.

- Stick to a generally low-cholesterol diet.
- Watch your carbohydrates. People with type 2 diabetes were put on a low-carb diet — only about 20 percent of their daily calories came from carbohydrates. After just six months, the chemical markers of inflammation in their blood were significantly lower than those on a low-fat diet.
- Get familiar with the glycemic index, a measure of how much individual foods increase the glucose in your blood. Experts believe a high-glycemic-load diet may stimulate inflammation.
- Avoid trans fat.
- Don't eat highly processed foods or charred or fried meat. They contain advanced glycation end products (AGEs), toxic chemicals formed in certain foods during cooking, processing, or packaging. If you get them in only small amounts, your body naturally eliminates them. In large quantities, however, they can build up and cause inflammation.

Mediterranean diet thrashes chronic disease

Eat delicious foods and stay healthy for life? It's a big promise, but the acclaimed Mediterranean diet may deliver.

This eating plan has its origins in regions surrounding the Mediterranean Sea, like Greece, Italy, and southern France. Here, traditional food and drinks are simple, natural, full of flavor, and above all, healthy.

As early as 1960, experts were intrigued by the low chronic disease rates and high life expectancies in this area. It seemed when all other factors were eliminated, diet was the only explanation. Although nutritionists may not agree on just one Mediterranean diet plan, all say you must have seven types of food in your diet if you want to lower your blood pressure, control blood sugar, rein in cholesterol, avoid cancer, and live longer.

- Whole-grains are the backbone of this diet. Naturally rich in fiber, vitamins, and minerals, you need several servings a day of brown rice, grains like barley and bulgur, whole oats, and breads or pasta made from whole-grain flour. These will fill you up, work to sweep your arteries clear of cholesterol, and fight a multitude of cancers.

- Fruits should become your new dessert. Naturally sweet, they can satisfy that sugar craving while still giving you a healthy dose of vitamins and minerals.

- Vegetables are vital to this diet. Fill half your plate with everything from artichokes to zucchini. It's hard to go wrong here, unless you deep-fry or slather them with butter and sauces.

- Nuts and seeds may surprise you with their health benefits. Rich in vitamin E, monounsaturated and polyunsaturated fats, fiber, and protein, they battle harmful inflammation behind chronic disease. Just remember they are heavy in calories, so watch your portions and eat them as a substitute for other fat sources. Use them in desserts and sauces or grab a handful for a crunchy snack.

- Beans and legumes provide fiber and other important nutrients without adding a lot of calories. Build a meal around them several times a week to help you cut back on the saturated fat in red meat.

- Olive oil could very well be called the elixir of life. It's that good for you. With almost 10 grams of monounsaturated fat and 103 milligrams of omega-3 fatty acids in every tablespoon, olive oil is considered a high-fat food. But, remember, these are healthy fats that fight heart disease and certain cancers. In addition, olive oil contains specific natural plant compounds, called phytochemicals, that act as antioxidants to fight damaging free radicals.

- Fish should be on your menu at least twice a week. Choose salmon, sardines, and tuna for their rich stores of heart-healthy, anti-inflammatory omega-3 fatty acids.

Add low-fat dairy and the occasional egg or chicken dish into the mix, and you have a nearly perfect approach to healthy eating. It's not rocket science. It doesn't involve going to a doctor, and it isn't even that hard to do. But it is full of variety and flavor and will help you fight chronic diseases.

Strip cancer of its power. What makes cancer cells so formidable is that they just won't die. These abnormal cells grow uncontrollably, forming masses that can invade healthy tissue and interfere with normal body processes like digestion, circulation, and your nervous system. Experts have discovered a compound in many foods of the Mediterranean diet that changes cancerous cells' behavior so they die normally. Research shows this diet is specifically helpful in combating breast, colon, oral, prostate, and skin cancers.

Strengthen your heart. Experts know exactly what is one driving force behind heart disease — inflammation. Reverse or prevent this inflammation, and you've just dealt heart disease a lethal blow. The Mediterranean diet, chock-full of inflammation-fighting compounds in fish, produce, whole grains, and olive oil, can do just that. A landmark Italian study of close to 15,000 adults found those on the Mediterranean diet tested with lower blood levels of two indicators of inflammation. Antioxidants, fiber, and the polyphenols in virgin olive oil are especially important to this benefit.

Other research showed people who most closely followed the Mediterranean diet had higher HDL (good) cholesterol and lower LDL (bad) cholesterol. This is one smart way you can practically guarantee flexible arteries for a lifetime.

Get serious diabetes protection. Whether you already suffer from diabetes or just want to safeguard yourself from its ravages, you'll want to "eat like a Greek." The Mediterranean diet can fight inflammation, oxidative stress, and insulin resistance, all factors that contribute to diabetes. Experts believe it's a combination of phytochemicals and minerals, plus a cutback in carbohydrates, that make this possible.

Need even more reasons to embrace this healthy way of eating? With it, you can manage your weight, ward off arthritis, fight depression, keep your brain sharp, and even protect it from Alzheimer's disease.

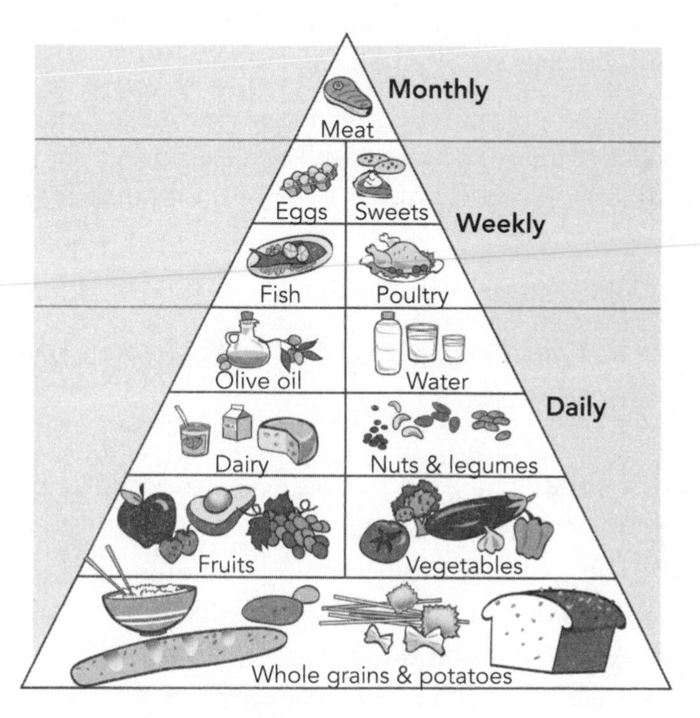

Mediterranean diet

Dodge a metabolic meltdown

It's a deadly combination of dangerous conditions, putting you at high risk of heart disease, diabetes, and stroke.

It's called metabolic syndrome and is fast becoming a global epidemic, with more than a third of adults affected in the United States alone.

You officially suffer from metabolic syndrome if you have three or more of the following:

- Abdominal obesity. A waist circumference of 40 inches or more in men, and 35 inches or more in women.
- High blood triglycerides. Levels of 150 milligrams per deciliter of blood (mg/dL) or higher.
- Low good cholesterol. Levels of HDL cholesterol below 40 mg/dL for men or 50 mg/dL for women.
- High blood pressure. Systolic blood pressure — the top number — more than 129 millimeters of mercury (mm Hg), or diastolic blood pressure — the bottom number — more than 84 mm Hg.
- High blood sugar. A fasting glucose of 100 mg/dL or greater.

While age and genetics play a small role in metabolic syndrome, you can take control of most risk factors with four simple lifestyle changes.

Drop extra pounds. Start with a modest 5 to 10 percent of your body weight, and you'll reduce your risks significantly. Aim to bring your body mass index (BMI) to below 25.

Stretch your legs. Melt belly fat, clear your arteries, improve blood pressure, and lower blood sugar, all by adding a brisk 30-minute walk to your daily routine. Regular exercise like this can prevent or manage metabolic syndrome and a host of other ailments. Plus you'll get an emotional lift and find you have more energy than you ever thought possible.

Make smart food choices. In the famous PREDIMED study out of Spain, people with metabolic syndrome following the Mediterranean diet were able to reverse the condition by improving two important symptoms — abdominal obesity and high blood sugar.

Take a test. Have your doctor routinely check your blood glucose and cholesterol levels. Stay on top of your blood pressure by monitoring it at home or at your local pharmacy.

Diabetes: outwit a deadly diagnosis

7 warning signs your body is headed for trouble

When are those annoying signs of aging in fact warnings of a bigger, nastier problem? Perhaps you've begun to have some trouble hearing, or you experience blurry vision, fatigue, or even more frequent trips to the bathroom. Everyone develops these issues as they get older, right? Not necessarily. Subtle changes like these could be symptoms of type 2 diabetes.

The reality is about 28 percent of people with diabetes are undiagnosed. More than 8 million individuals in the United States are walking around with this potentially deadly disease and don't know it. So just what is going on in your body?

Beware prediabetes. First, let's start with glucose, or blood sugar. It most often comes from foods you eat and is the major source of energy for all the cells in your body. It travels in your bloodstream but can't actually enter cells without the help of insulin, a hormone made in your pancreas by special beta cells. The trouble starts when you make enough insulin, but for some reason, your body doesn't let it do its job and all the glucose in your blood can't get into your cells. This is called insulin resistance — your cells "resist" the insulin. It takes extra insulin for even some of the glucose to get absorbed.

Now it becomes a vicious cycle. Your cells need energy but can't absorb all the glucose. Your pancreas gets the message to make even more insulin. As long as the beta cells can keep up with this extra demand, your glucose levels remain normal. But eventually they fail, and glucose begins to build up in your bloodstream. You are now one of the 86 million people in the U.S. who suffer from prediabetes, a condition where blood glucose levels are higher than normal. This also means you are at a higher risk of developing full-blown type 2 diabetes and heart disease.

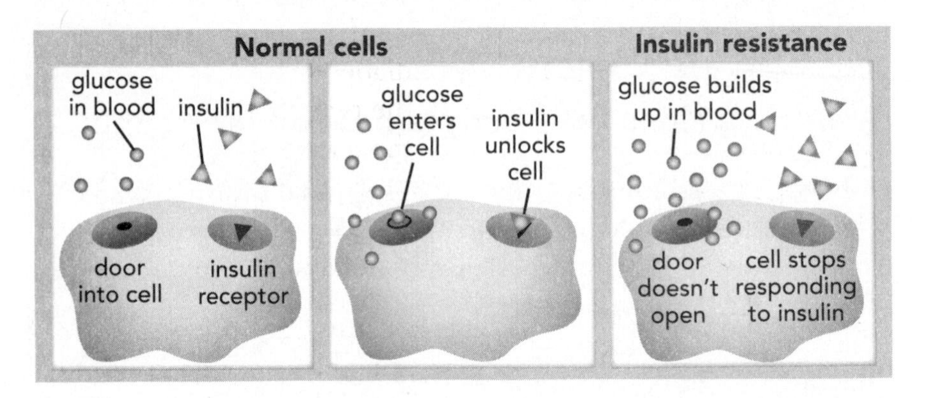

Don't ignore these symptoms. But let's return to those missed signs. How are they related to diabetes?

- Blurred vision and hearing problems. Glucose that builds up in your blood can distort the lens in your eye, changing its shape and causing things to look unfocused. It may also damage the nerves and small blood vessels in your inner ear.
- Fatigue. Of course you're tired. Your cells aren't getting enough glucose for the energy you need.
- Frequent urination. This is your body's attempt to get rid of all that extra glucose. When you go to the bathroom often you may also become dehydrated and feel thirsty all the time.

There are other warning signs you shouldn't disregard. If you're constantly hungry, your body could be trying to provide your cells with the energy they need, but aren't getting. Patches of darkened skin on your neck, knuckles, or in fat folds are caused by excess pigment stimulated by insulin. And if you notice tingling or numbness in your hands and feet, or have cuts that don't heal, your blood vessels and nerves may be damaged from too much glucose. All these could signal prediabetes or diabetes.

Get on the scale. Hands down, being overweight is the greatest risk factor for diabetes. The obesity epidemic of the past two decades has driven up the threat of diabetes in the U.S. from 20 percent to over 40 percent. In fact, the two conditions are so closely related, experts have coined the term "diabesity." Fat, especially belly fat, is more inflammatory than other types of cells and can set in motion the changes that lead to diabetes. Fat cells also produce certain hormones that trigger insulin resistance.

Recognize your risk. While you can control lifestyle behaviors that contribute to diabetes, such as eating habits, physical activity, and smoking, you can't change certain risk factors like genetics, age, sex, and ethnicity. Hispanics and African-Americans are at greater risk, for instance.

Experts have also noticed that people with sleep apnea or gout are more likely to develop diabetes. And if you have a high-stress job, do shift work, or routinely have a work week of greater than 55 hours, especially at manual labor, you're more likely to develop diabetes.

Understand, these factors don't actually cause diabetes but may indicate you are at higher risk. If they apply to you, talk to your doctor.

Take aim against diabetes' deadly dangers

Diabetes is called the silent killer for a reason. Most of the complications from this disease won't become evident until 10 to 15 years after your initial diagnosis. If you aren't proactive right away, in 10 years you could be knee-deep in dangerous, possibly life-threatening, consequences.

Heart disease. Half the people with diabetes die of heart disease. That's an alarming statistic. Not only that, but it's likely you'll develop heart disease at a far younger age than people without diabetes. Why is this so?

- Because you're insulin resistant, you've got extra glucose in your blood, which damages the lining of your arteries. Fatty deposits, called plaque, build up in these damaged areas, harden over time, and narrow the arteries. Blood has a harder time flowing through these narrow, stiff arteries. Clots often form, further obstructing blood flow, and often break free to cause a heart attack.
- New research proposes an additional theory. Again the culprit is excess blood sugar, which may cause microscopic damage to your heart muscle. "It looks like diabetes may be slowly killing heart muscle in ways we had not thought of before," says Dr. Elizabeth Selvin, the study's leader.

Vision loss. The retina is a layer of cells at the back of your eyeball that sends images to your brain. Long-term damage to the tiny blood vessels here means they can bulge, leak, or even rupture. You may know it as diabetic retinopathy. Depending on the severity of the damage, you could experience blurriness or temporary, even permanent blindness.

Kidney damage. Your kidneys are remarkable organs — ones you literally can't live without. Their job is to filter waste material from your blood and flush it out of your body through your urine. It's an amazingly elegant and complex system.

When you have high levels of sugar in your blood, your kidneys must work extra hard to filter out impurities. After years of this strain, they become less efficient. Useful substances like protein and red blood cells get passed into your urine, and waste products remain in your blood. Eventually, your kidneys fail completely and you must have a kidney transplant or have your blood filtered by a dialysis machine.

Nerve damage. When the nerves throughout your body are damaged by too much blood sugar, it is called diabetic neuropathy and can affect you in ways you never imagined.

- Peripheral neuropathy targets your feet and hands. You'll experience pain, tingling, burning, or numbness. You may even have trouble walking.
- Autonomic neuropathy can involve your bladder, digestive system, sweat glands, sex organs, and more. Any or all of these systems may stop functioning properly.

Memory loss. Diabetes is not good for your brain. In fact, you're twice as likely as people without diabetes to suffer memory loss or some other kind of mental impairment, particularly if you're middle-aged.

- Damage to the blood vessels that deliver nutrients to your brain means you could suffer ministrokes that trigger dementia.
- Blood sugar levels that yo-yo from extreme highs to sudden lows are very damaging to brain cells, with experts actually calling the effects of sugar "toxic." Researchers specializing in neuroradiology studied over 600 people with diabetes. They noticed shrinking in their brains, especially in areas that control muscles, vision, memory, emotions, and speech. The longer the people had diabetes, the worse the damage.

Cancer. Both the American Diabetes Association and the American Cancer Society feel the relationship between diabetes and cancer needs to be explored further. Evidence suggests you have a higher risk of colon, breast, bladder, liver, pancreas, and endometrial cancers if you have diabetes.

It may simply be that the conditions share common risk factors, such as obesity, poor diet, and lack of exercise. Or it could be the cancers are triggered by high levels of insulin, blood sugar, or inflammation associated with diabetes. Be sure you are screened for these and other cancers.

In addition, if you have diabetes, you may develop foot ulcers, skin problems, nonalcoholic fatty liver disease, gum disease, and depression. The good news is you can prevent or limit the progression of most of these complications by keeping your blood sugar on an even keel. Get the correct medical treatment and make the healthy changes you'll read about next — embrace smart diet choices, take natural supplements, and engage in healthy activities.

Nutritional know-how tames blood sugar

Three simple things can help you reverse the effects of type 2 diabetes — eating healthy, getting regular physical activity, and losing weight. The first thing to focus on is your diet, or nutrition therapy, as experts sometimes call it.

- The goal, if you are at risk of diabetes, is to better your odds. Start right now making some generally smart food choices — increase fruits, vegetables, and whole grains while eliminating saturated fats and sugary drinks — and you could reduce your risk by 20 percent, compared to people who don't change their diets.
- If you already have diabetes, the goal is to get your blood sugar, blood pressure, and cholesterol numbers within healthy limits; reach a healthy weight; and prevent or delay the complications of diabetes. At the same time you need foods that will fuel your body and you will enjoy eating. That's quite a challenge, especially since experts agree there is no one-size-fits-all diet.

  Their best advice? Concentrate on quality rather than quantity — high-quality fats and high-quality carbs. Then choose an eating plan that fits your lifestyle and food preferences. You could start with the anti-inflammatory diet or the Mediterranean diet you read about in the chapter *Inflammation: stamp out the source of disease.*

Finally, meet with a registered dietitian for help with meal planning and portion control. In addition, here are some other changes you could make.

Cut your carbs. Many experts believe diabetes is all about carbohydrates — more specifically, how your body responds to them. Carbs, which include sugars as well as grains, have a huge impact on your weight and the amount of glucose in your blood. A low-carbohydrate diet can be a real cure for many people with type 2 diabetes, says Barbara Gower, Ph.D., professor and vice chair for research in the Department of Nutrition Sciences at the University of Alabama at Birmingham. "They no longer need drugs. They no longer have symptoms. Their blood glucose is normal, and they generally lose weight."

While the 2010 Dietary Guidelines for Americans recommends 45 to 65 percent of your daily calories come from carbohydrates, the numbers behind a low-carb diet may be confusing. Here are some definitions approved by experts in nutrition research. Talk to your doctor to find out what number is right for you.

Carbohydrate grams per day (based on a 2,000-calorie-per-day diet)	
Very-low-carbohydrate diet	20 - 50
Low-carbohydrate diet	50 - 130
Moderate-carbohydrate diet	130 - 225
High-carbohydrate diet	more than 225

Bump up your fiber. Want an amazing fun fact about fiber? You don't digest it. That means it can't raise the level of glucose in your blood. But it can stabilize, even lower it in a rather roundabout way. Fiber slows down digestion and carbohydrate absorption, which means it can reduce your cholesterol and cause fewer blood sugar spikes after eating. In short, more fiber means better glycemic control. Indulge your sweet tooth with high-fiber dried fruits, berries, apples, and guavas.

Improve vitamin D levels. If you're prediabetic and have a low amount of vitamin D in your body, taking a supplement could improve your blood sugar. A two-year study out of India found glucose levels returned to normal for twice as many people taking vitamin D as those in the group without supplements. The researchers believe the vitamin battles insulin resistance and inflammation. Have your doctor check your levels of vitamin D and advise you about supplements.

Can glycemic index help contol blood sugar?

Your body burns sugar like your car burns gas, and carbohydrates are your main source of this fuel. Different carbs break down into glucose — or sugar — at different rates, depending on their structure. Some burn quickly, releasing a flood of glucose into your bloodstream. To counter that, your body needs to release a large amount of insulin. Other carbohydrates take longer to digest, giving you a slower, steadier supply of glucose.

The glycemic index (GI) measures a food's ability to raise your blood sugar and ranks it from 0 to 100. Slower-burning foods have a low GI value of 0 to 55, medium GIs are 56 to 69, and fast-burning, high-GI foods rank from 70 to 100. For reference, pure glucose has a GI value of 100.

Just as the slow and steady tortoise beat the speedy hare in the famous fable, slow-burning carbohydrates have the advantage when it comes to your health. Eating low-GI foods can help keep your insulin, your blood sugar, and your appetite steady.

Several factors affect a food's GI rating, including fat and fiber content, ripeness of fruits and vegetables, amount of processing, and cooking method.

High-GI foods	Low-GI substitutions
white potatoes	sweet potatoes, lentils, beans
crackers, pretzels, pastries	whole-grain bars, fresh or dried fruit, nuts
processed cereals	old-fashioned oats or muesli
jasmine and arborio rice	long-grain or basmati rice, pasta, quinoa
sodas	fruit juices or low-fat milk
hard candy	raisins or a piece of chocolate
white bread	whole-grain, sourdough, or pumpernickel
sugar	honey

The glycemic index alone does not account for portion size. You can choose all low-GI foods, but if you eat too many of them, you will still end up overweight and battling high blood sugar. That's where the glycemic load (GL) comes in. To figure out GL, you need to know the GI value of a food as well as its available carbohydrates per serving — total carbs minus fiber. Multiply the two numbers together and divide the result by 100. Generally, a GL below 10 is considered low; above 20 is considered high.

The glycemic index and glycemic load are valuable tools to help control your blood sugar levels. Unfortunately, they can also be hard to follow. Use handy GI and GL food lists to guide you to the right choices. Or search for the GI and GL of specific foods for free at the website *www.glycemicindex.com*.

10 superfoods that can change your life

The American Diabetes Association has come up with its own list of 10 superfoods. All have a low glycemic index yet are rich in nutrients important to those suffering from diabetes. Work them into your menu whenever possible.

Superfood	Nutritional benefit
beans	packed with fiber, magnesium, and potassium; a cheap source of protein
berries	bursting with antioxidants, fiber, and vitamins
citrus	a sweet way to get soluble fiber and vitamin C
green leafy vegetables	chock-full of vitamins yet low in carbohydrates and calories
fat-free dairy	boosts your intake of vitamin D
nuts	controls hunger while providing omega-3 fatty acids, magnesium, and fiber
salmon	rich in omega-3 fatty acids
sweet potatoes	filled with fiber and beta carotene
tomatoes	provides lycopene, iron, vitamin C, and vitamin A
whole grains	crammed with fiber plus extra vitamins and minerals through enrichment

Make the right choice: supplements that fight diabetes

Diabetes is serious business. That's why the Food and Drug Administration (FDA) is cracking down on products and treatments that promise to prevent and even cure the disease. Not only can they contain unsafe ingredients, but if you take them instead of seeking real medical care, you could be putting your life at risk.

Experts do consider some over-the-counter supplements safe, however. You may have already read about fish oil supplements for inflammation in the chapter *Fats: the ones to pick, the ones to pitch*. Here are some others you and your doctor could consider.

- A good multivitamin and mineral supplement is a form of dietary insurance most people should take.

- Alpha-lipoic acid may improve insulin sensitivity, blood sugar control, and symptoms of peripheral neuropathy.
- American ginseng (*Panax quinquefolium*) can reduce blood sugar spikes and fasting blood glucose levels.
- Beta-glucan is a type of soluble fiber proven to lower cholesterol and control blood sugar.
- Magnesium helps your body break down sugars and might lower your risk of insulin resistance.

Tap into the healing power of fitness

Being overweight is the number one risk factor for type 2 diabetes. And the heavier you are, the greater your risk. Is that enough to get you off the couch? Just consider the rewards.

If you have prediabetes and commit to boosting your physical activity just a little — say a 30-minute brisk walk five days a week — and dropping at least a few pounds, you could cut your risk for full-blown diabetes in half.

But what if you already have diabetes? Simple lifestyle changes like these could:

- get your blood sugar levels under control. Remember, glucose is energy. So when you're active, your body naturally uses it up. That means less glucose in your bloodstream triggering insulin production and wreaking other kinds of havoc.
- lower your blood pressure, cholesterol, and your risk of a devastating heart attack within the next five years.
- reduce your healthcare costs on average by more than $500 a year.

Getting fit must be a lifelong strategy. So be safe and smart. Start slowly, with your doctor's supervision. Try a combination of walking and weight training for best results.

- Work toward an hour alternating between walking rapidly for three minutes then at a slower pace for three minutes. In studies, this controlled blood sugar better than walking at a constant pace. In fact, walking is so good for your glucose levels and body weight, it can reduce your need for diabetes medications.
- Lifting weights increases your muscle mass, burns calories, uses up glucose, helps you lose weight, and fights insulin resistance.

Good reason to rethink that diet soda

What if, with every sip of a sugar-free soda or bite of a diet snack, artificial sweeteners were actually setting you up for blood sugar spikes?

Scientists, reporting on a new study in the journal *Nature*, discovered sweeteners like saccharin, sucralose, and aspartame changed the digestive tract bacteria in some people so they became glucose intolerant, a condition related to insulin resistance and a risk factor for developing type 2 diabetes.

No doubt about it, stepping away from that diet soda is not a bad thing, overall. And chemical sweeteners have come under fire in the past because of potential health risks. But every person has a unique blend of gut bacteria and so may respond differently to foods and additives.

Your best bet? Stay tuned for more, larger studies on this potential danger, and, in the meantime, dial down your sugar intake by limiting foods that are either naturally or artificially sweetened.

Heart disease: attack the #1 killer

Positive steps to a healthy heart

Your heart works harder than any other muscle in your body. It's not the longest. That distinction belongs to the muscle in your thigh. It's not the strongest. Surprisingly, your jaw muscle wins that prize. And it's not the largest. You're probably sitting on that one right now. But it is the hardest-working, every day beating about 100,000 times and pumping almost 2,000 gallons of blood throughout your body.

Even though it's the power behind the very essence of life, this fist-size muscle is unexpectedly fragile. So much can go wrong. And when it does, it's usually disastrous. Heart disease is the leading cause of death in the United States, for both men and women, killing over 600,000 people every year. The real tragedy is one-third of those could have been prevented just by changing habits and managing health risks.

The peril that is plaque. Ground zero for heart disease is plaque. As you read in the *Inflammation: stamp out the source of disease* chapter, microscopic damage to the inner lining of your arteries allows tiny cholesterol particles to clump, forming a waxy buildup called plaque. Over time, plaque can harden, then narrow and even block your arteries. This condition is called atherosclerosis or coronary heart disease (CHD).

Complications that can kill. Once you develop CHD, you're vulnerable to a host of related complications.

- Angina pectoris. This brief episode of pain can feel like a giant hand is squeezing your chest. The discomfort can even extend to your arms, back, neck, or jaw. It's triggered during exercise or times of stress, when your heart is working harder than normal but can't get enough blood because of blocked arteries.

- Unstable angina. Compared to angina pectoris, the pain is more severe, lasts longer — often more than 20 minutes — and isn't eased with rest or medication. Unstable angina can lead to a heart attack, so consider it an emergency situation.

- Heart failure. Over time, CHD damages your heart so much it can no longer pump strongly enough to circulate the blood your body needs. You'll feel tired, find it difficult to breathe, and start retaining fluid in your lungs, feet, and ankles. You'll need to change your diet, start exercising, take medications, and perhaps consider surgery.

- Arrhythmia. Any time you have an ongoing problem with the rate or rhythm of your heartbeat, you suffer from arrhythmia. Atrial fibrillation or AFib is the most common serious type of arrhythmia in people over age 65. There's a variety of causes behind AFib, but regardless, it increases your risk of heart attack and stroke. Reduce the threat by controlling your blood pressure, cholesterol, and weight.

Changes that can save your life. Heart disease has reached epidemic proportions largely due to today's lifestyle — sitting in a car, recliner, or computer chair with a cheeseburger in one hand and a soda in the other. The American Heart Association believes there are several simple steps you can take to improve your overall health and cut your risk of heart disease.

- get active
- lose weight
- control cholesterol
- reduce blood sugar
- eat better
- stop smoking
- manage blood pressure

Read about them in the following stories, as well as other sections of this book.

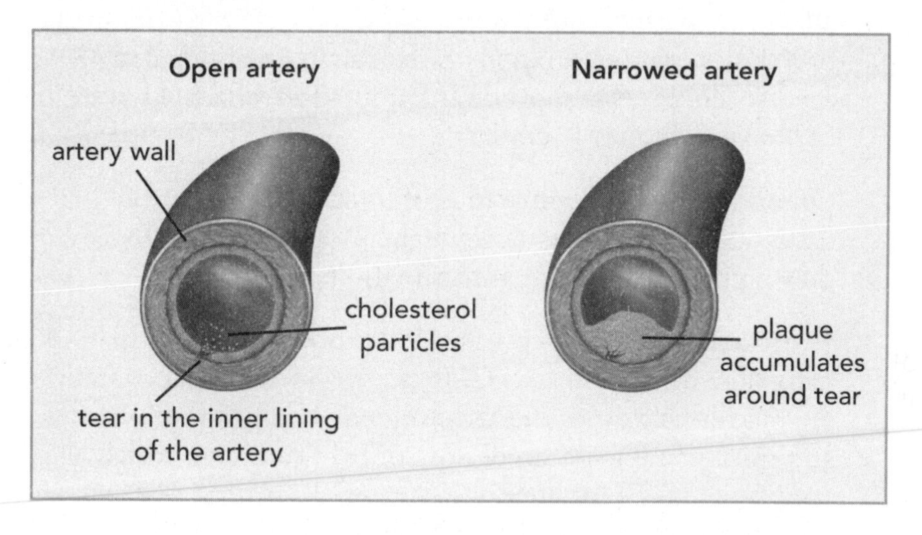

Sofrito: a nutritious treat for body and soul

Separately, each ingredient is a healthy home run. But combine tomatoes, onions, garlic, peppers, and olive oil into a tasty sauce known as sofrito, and you've just hit a grand slam of flavor and wellness.

Foodies may debate the finer points of preparation and origin — variations show up in Portuguese, Cuban, Spanish, and Latin American cuisines — but there's no arguing how good sofrito is for you. All the ingredients contain vitamins, minerals, and naturally occurring plant chemicals that battle chronic conditions like heart disease and cancer.

- Tomatoes, in any form, fight heart disease, stroke, and high blood pressure. They are loaded with lycopene, a phytochemical that fends off cell-damaging toxins, improves cholesterol and triglyceride levels, plus reduces inflammation. Eat your tomatoes cooked, or even processed into paste, sauce, soup, or juice, and the lycopene power is even greater.

- Garlic may be one of the world's healthiest foods. It contains more than 2,000 compounds that can, in various ways, affect cells within your body. Most notably, garlic can lower bad cholesterol, relax blood vessels, act as an antioxidant against cancer cells, suppress inflammation, and fight even antibiotic-resistant bacteria.
- Onions are an excellent source of fiber, folic acid, antioxidants, and the important phytochemical quercetin. Together they battle heart disease, inflammation, and cancer.
- Sweet red and green peppers may surprise you with their hefty dose of vitamin C — a single, small red pepper contains one-and-a-half times the recommended daily amount. In addition, you'll get a super dose of beta carotene, which your body needs for good vision, to fight cancer, and to protect your brain against decline.

To make approximately two cups of sofrito, coarsely chop one green pepper, one red pepper, two medium tomatoes, one medium onion, and three to four garlic cloves. Heat one-fourth to one-half cup virgin olive oil in a saucepan, then add the vegetables. Simmer, stirring occasionally, for about 30 minutes. Serve as a sauce or garnish on meat, vegetables, or eggs.

3 ways to cut cholesterol confusion

Cholesterol isn't all bad. In fact, your liver makes about 1,000 milligrams of this soft, waxy substance a day. On purpose. Your cells need it to maintain their structure, create hormones, convert sunlight into vitamin D, and produce bile acids that help digest fat.

Crack the cholesterol code. To get to all your cells, cholesterol must travel in your bloodstream. But since it's a type of fat and your blood is mostly water, the two don't mix. So the cholesterol hitches a ride on protein molecules. These little protein-cholesterol packages are called lipoproteins. The amount of protein molecules in each varies and is referred to as density.

- Low-density lipoproteins (LDLs) have fewer protein molecules and are the major cholesterol carriers in your blood. If there are lots of them circulating, that means your cells don't need any more cholesterol and have locked the doors, so to speak. The LDLs stay in your bloodstream, dumping their extra cholesterol onto your artery walls willy-nilly. There it clumps and forms dangerous plaque, a condition called atherosclerosis. LDLs are often called "bad" cholesterol, but they are really only harmful when you have too many of them. A high blood level of LDL cholesterol usually means you also have more of a fatty buildup in your arteries.
- High-density lipoproteins (HDLs) are considered the good guys because they clean up excess cholesterol and carry it back to your liver where it gets flushed out of your body.

Often, in addition to cholesterol, lipoproteins will transport a common type of fat called triglycerides. Those that carry the most triglycerides and the least amount of protein are called very low-density lipoproteins (VLDLs). Having high VLDL levels means you not only have lots of cholesterol in your bloodstream but lots of dangerous fat cells, too.

Gauge your total risk. You can have high cholesterol and not know it. That's why it's so important to get regular blood tests to check your levels. From a "lipoprotein profile," you'll find out your total cholesterol, LDL, HDL, and triglyceride numbers. They are measured as milligrams of cholesterol per deciliter of blood, or mg/dL.

That said, many experts, including the American Heart Association and the American College of Cardiology, are abandoning the long-held "know your number" campaign. They recently published new heart attack and stroke prevention guidelines that focus on a total package of lifestyle, obesity, risk assessment, and cholesterol recommendations — sort of a "know your risk" campaign. Their Risk Calculator, which you can find by searching on the American Heart Association's website at *http://my.americanheart.org*, factors in age, sex, race, cholesterol and blood pressure numbers, current health, and smoking history to compute your 10-year risk of heart disease and stroke.

Reassess the numbers. As far as cholesterol levels are concerned, these same organizations say unless you have very high cholesterol, chasing a specific number does not always mean a lower risk of heart disease. You may use medication to get your numbers to an acceptable level, but if you haven't addressed other factors, such as weight, diet, and exercise, you may feel a false sense of security. Along those same lines, don't let a good HDL number overshadow a bad LDL number. Any high non-HDL number is dangerous.

That's why the traditional method of figuring LDL cholesterol, called the Friedewald Equation, is being challenged. Here's an example of this, where total cholesterol is 220, HDL is 50, and triglycerides are 150.

Total cholesterol	220
HDL cholesterol	- 50
	170
Triglycerides 150 ÷ 5	- 30
LDL cholesterol	140

As you can see, this calculation gives an LDL reading of 140 that falls in the "Borderline" category. Researchers at the Johns Hopkins University School of Medicine think you get a more accurate assessment of artery health if you leave dangerous triglycerides in the calculation. They propose an alternate method, resulting in a higher, non-HDL level. In this example, the number 170 places you squarely in the "Dangerous" category.

	Total Cholesterol	LDL (bad) Cholesterol	HDL (good) Cholesterol
Dangerous	>240	>160	<40
Borderline	200-239	100-160	
Healthy	<200	<100	>60

Stop high cholesterol in its tracks

You don't need more cholesterol than your body makes naturally. Yet some people are genetically predisposed to make too much and others produce extra during certain times of their lives. In addition, you may be making diet and lifestyle choices that cause dangerous increases in your cholesterol levels. Even so, you have the power to fix the problem.

Choose a healthy menu. What you eat affects the amount of cholesterol in your body. Specific heart-healthy eating plans like the Mediterranean Diet focus on fruits, vegetables, whole grains, and good fats. Read about it in other sections of this book. You can also make some food choices that will improve your cholesterol levels.

- Avoid saturated fats found in meats and full-fat dairy, trans fats in hard margarines and commercial baked goods, added sugars, and fructose-sweetened drinks and other foods.

- Choose oils carefully. Stay away from palm oil, coconut oil, and cocoa butter. The polyunsaturated fats found in corn, sunflower, and walnut oil, however, are proven to be especially helpful in lowering LDL levels.
- Bump up the amount of soluble fiber in your diet. This kind ferments in your large intestines, producing a short-chain fatty acid that limits how much cholesterol your liver produces. It also sweeps up bile as it passes through your digestive system and carries it out of your body, triggering a series of events that cause your liver to pull even more LDL cholesterol out of your blood. The National Cholesterol Education Program encourages you to increase your daily intake of soluble fiber to 10 to 25 grams a day. Good choices are oatmeal, lentils, apples, oranges, strawberries, nuts, dried beans and peas, blueberries, celery, and carrots.
- Boost the amount of monounsaturated fat (MUFA) you eat by choosing foods like avocados and nuts, proven to lower bad cholesterol levels. Surprisingly, eggs fall into this healthy category, with 38 percent of their fat being the monounsaturated kind. One test of a high-egg diet — 140 overweight people ate two eggs a day, six days a week, for three months — even showed improvement in HDL levels.

Ditch extra pounds. Those pesky fat cells are sabotaging your efforts to stay healthy. Scientists have discovered they produce a protein, called resistin, that not only prompts liver cells to produce more LDLs but then blocks cholesterol-lowering drugs, like statins, from working properly. The result — a pileup of bad cholesterol in your arteries. And if you're overweight, your HDL cholesterol levels tend to be lower.

Experts say lose just 10 percent of your body weight and you can set things right. You'll not only lower your cholesterol, blood pressure, and risk of heart disease, but reap other healthy rewards, as well.

Get physical. Must you work out like a demon to clear your arteries? Experts say no. Moderate activity like brisk walking is just as good for lowering cholesterol levels as running, and you're less likely to hurt yourself. If you can't dedicate hours out of your day to getting fit, think small. A short burst of activity, less than 10 minutes, was proven to be just as beneficial as a longer session. Whatever you do, just make it a regular habit.

Take a chill pill. Emotional stress, especially from a high-pressure job, changes the way your body balances fat levels in your blood. A Scandinavian study of 90,000 workers found those with high job stress were more likely to have too much LDL cholesterol and abnormally low amounts of HDL cholesterol. Offset your workday stress with exercise or relaxing activities like yoga or massage, listening to music, or watching a funny movie.

Pick up a probiotic. Your body contains trillions of bacteria. The good bacteria keep you healthy by fighting infections, digesting your food, producing vitamins, and more. To give your unique colony of bacteria a boost, you can take a supplement of live bacteria, called a probiotic. Different probiotics contain varying strains of bacteria that are known to do different things. The strain *Lactobacillus reuteri* NCIMB 30242 was shown in studies to lower blood levels of LDL cholesterol by almost 12 percent in just nine weeks. Experts believe it works by breaking up bile salts, thus limiting how much cholesterol is absorbed in your gut.

Supplement with B5. Pantethine, a form of vitamin B5 or pantothenic acid, may be one natural way you can improve your cholesterol levels. A recent, small study showed that 600 to 900 milligrams of pantethine a day for four months lowered dangerous LDL levels by 11 percent. This supplement has been used safely in Japan for decades, and multiple trials have shown no major side effects. To be on the safe side, always talk to your doctor before you take any supplement.

Beware hidden cholesterol hazards

Cholesterol can clog your arteries and cause life-threatening clots. But it's also linked to other serious health problems.

- Very early research suggests a byproduct of cholesterol metabolism acts like estrogen to fuel and spread the growth of breast cancer cells.
- Unhealthy levels of cholesterol are linked to brain amyloid plaques, an indicator of Alzheimer's disease.
- Even before you're diagnosed with diabetes, any degree of insulin resistance fouls up your cholesterol levels. Your HDL levels drop and LDL numbers increase, a condition called diabetic dyslipidemia.

Statins: miracle cure or dangerous drug?

Should you take a pill every day for the rest of your life to stay healthy? Two hundred million people worldwide do. That's how many are prescribed statins — a class of drugs that dramatically lowers cholesterol, thus cutting heart attack and stroke risk anywhere from 20 to 50 percent. As good as that sounds, the debate over the risks versus the benefits of statins is not new.

Diabetes. Taking a statin can increase your risk of developing type 2 diabetes, perhaps by raising your blood sugar, interfering with insulin production, or by causing you to gain weight. Experts call it a "modest" increase in risk but say it mostly pertains to people who take statins for a long time, are prescribed high-powered versions or high doses, or already have other diabetes risk factors.

Offsetting this not-so-good news, a Danish study of more than 60,000 people with diabetes found those who were already taking statins before being diagnosed with the disease developed fewer complications, like nerve and eye damage, within a three-year followup.

Weight gain. A 12-year study has confirmed what millions suspect — taking a statin often means you'll gain weight. However, experts are quick to say, don't blame the drug since it doesn't seem to fiddle with your metabolism or your appetite. Many people on statins simply eat more, thinking the drug gives them a free pass to indulge. Over the course of this study, the statin users increased their calories by 9 percent and fat intake by 14 percent, while nonusers remained about the same.

In addition, liver damage used to be a major concern for statin users, but since 2012, the Food and Drug Administration (FDA) found it to be such a rare complication, they no longer recommend regular liver enzyme testing. And while there are other widespread side effects, including fatigue, muscle pain, and memory loss or confusion, 90 percent of the people in a recent study found a different statin or a lower dose worked for them without these complications.

While many experts believe the benefits of taking a statin outweigh the potential risks, the bottom line is you need to be an active participant in your own health care. Discuss your risks with your doctor, and if you decide to take a statin, step up your exercise routine and watch your diet.

High blood pressure: save your heart from the big squeeze

Every time your heart contracts, it pushes blood into your arteries. This period of time is known as systole. Then your heart relaxes, fills up with blood, and prepares to contract again. This is called diastole. The force, or pressure, of the blood in your arteries rises and falls as your heart contracts and relaxes. A blood pressure reading is the level of pressure during systole over the level of pressure during diastole, expressed in millimeters (mm) of mercury (Hg). The American Heart Association defines normal blood pressure as 120/80 mm Hg.

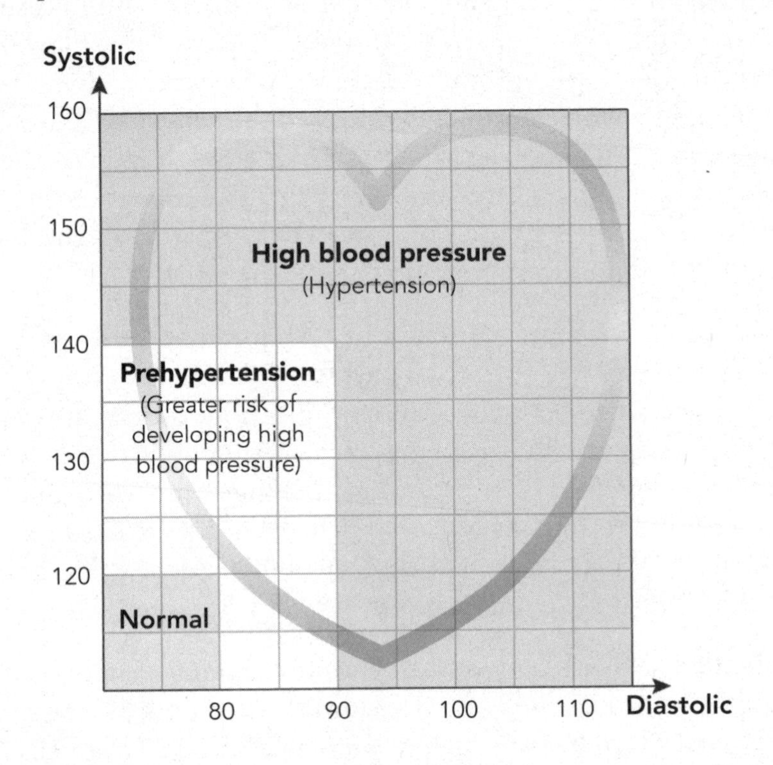

Something as healthy as exercise can cause a temporary increase in blood pressure by making your heart beat faster and harder to ferry extra oxygen and nutrients to your muscles. On the other hand, less healthy things can cause ongoing high blood pressure, like:

- plaque buildup on your artery walls that narrows and stiffens them.
- poorly functioning kidneys that can't rid your body of excess sodium.
- hormone abnormalities.

Untreated high blood pressure, or hypertension, can:

- damage your arteries so they rupture and cause a stroke or aneurysm.
- restrict life-giving blood and oxygen traveling to your tissues and organs.
- make your heart work even harder to force blood throughout your body.
- continue the dangerous cycle of high cholesterol and plaque buildup.

Drug-free ways to put the brakes on soaring blood pressure

You're at greater risk for strokes, heart attacks, vision loss, and kidney failure when your blood pressure is high. The good news is if you're committed to making some lifestyle changes, you can get this dangerous condition under control.

Let the sun shine in. As little as 20 minutes exposed to ultraviolet A (UVA) rays from the sun could lower your blood pressure. These rays trigger production of nitric oxide (NO), a compound that dilates and relaxes blood vessels. Experts believe the heart benefits of this short-term exposure outweigh any risk of skin cancer. Studies have also shown a relationship between higher vitamin D levels and lower blood pressure. Since you make vitamin D when your skin is exposed to the sun, a little natural light could help in this way, too.

Break the sugar habit. Sugar may be your blood vessels' new worst enemy. It affects the part of your brain that speeds up your heart rate and lowers your levels of NO, causing your blood vessels to constrict and your blood pressure to rise. When studies focused on people who regularly drank sugar-sweetened beverages or fruit juices high in natural sugars, they found they had significantly higher blood pressure than others.

Adopt man's best friend. Owning a dog can lower your blood pressure, your heart rate, and your stress levels. It may be the daily walks that do the trick, because dog owners usually have lower cholesterol levels and a lower rate of obesity, benefits also associated with regular exercise.

Take a probiotic. The good bacteria that keep your digestive system operating smoothly may have a hidden benefit — lower blood pressure. After looking at several studies, experts suggest you could get a modest drop in your systolic and diastolic numbers if you consume probiotics in fermented dairy products, like yogurt, or take them as a supplement for at least two months. The benefit was greatest among people with blood pressure over 130/85 mm Hg and if there were multiple strains of bacteria in the probiotics.

Give of your time. Doing a little good seems to do your heart a little good, too. Older people who volunteered a mere four hours every week were 40 percent less likely to develop high blood pressure four years later than those who didn't volunteer. It may be volunteering allows you to enjoy friendships and develop social connections, which lower your risk of high blood pressure. Or, since many volunteer opportunities require at least a little physical activity, it could be simply getting off the couch helps your heart. Others feel volunteers develop better coping mechanisms that combat stress and heart-damaging stress hormones.

Hold the salt. Whether you shake it on at the table or get it from processed foods, this combination of sodium and chloride can raise your blood pressure in two ways. First, it makes you retain water, which produces a greater volume of blood in your arteries. Then it constricts those arteries, causing your heart to work extra hard to pump blood throughout your body.

There's no doubt about it, most Americans get way too much salt — about 4,000 milligrams (mg) a day. Yet the American Heart Association recommends a daily quota of less than 1,500 mg, or just over half a teaspoon. Most experts agree the older you are and the higher your blood pressure, the more important salt levels are.

Keep tabs on your numbers. People with high blood pressure who regularly monitor it themselves tend to have lower numbers than people who don't track it at home. There are a few guidelines to getting the best readings.

- Buy a monitor with an arm cuff that automatically inflates.
- Make sure the cuff fits you. If it's too small or too large, your reading will be off.
- Take your monitor in to your doctor's office to check its accuracy against their machine.
- Check the pressure in both arms for a few days to see if they differ. Tell your doctor if one arm is consistently higher than the other, since it could mean you're at higher risk for other heart problems.
- Take a couple of readings a few minutes apart at random times during the day.
- Log your numbers into a notebook and take it to your next doctor's appointment. You'll get the most benefit if the two of you discuss the readings.

Bust the belly fat. Your weight is the single most important risk factor for high blood pressure you can change. And any extra pounds you carry around your middle magnifies that risk.

An exercise routine doesn't have to be excessive — aim for half an hour a day. Start by simply getting out of your chair. You can lower your systolic blood pressure just by breaking up long periods of sitting with a little exercise — take a walk or go for a swim. Working out in warm water dilates your blood vessels and improves blood flow, making it a great way to get fit and relax.

5 heart-saving strategies every woman must know

It's not just a "man's problem" anymore. Heart disease now affects and kills more women in the United States than men. So why is it that you, as a woman, are at a higher risk?

- You suffer more from certain autoimmune disorders, like rheumatoid arthritis and lupus, that are linked with a higher risk of heart disease.
- Specific conditions unique to women can increase your risk, like gestational diabetes, preeclampsia, and hormonal changes.
- You're more likely to ignore signs of heart disease because you feel your priority is taking care of others. Delayed care means the disease often progresses to the point where there are fewer treatment options.
- Experts say women don't usually react quickly or decisively to symptoms, instead chalking them up to some other, less dangerous, health condition, then talking to friends or family members about them instead of calling for professional help.
- You don't always receive the complete preventive guidance that men do, such as ways to lower your cholesterol, information on aspirin therapy, or lifestyle advice.
- You're not taking serious control of your own health. Based on data from the National Health and Nutrition Examination Survey, less than 2 percent of the almost 23,000 women surveyed embraced all seven of the American Heart Association's heart-saving lifestyle recommendations.

- Your coronary arteries are smaller in diameter than men's, which makes them more prone to blockages.

So first, make the changes you read about earlier in this chapter. Then try these other ways to keep from becoming a statistic.

Tame your temper. Mental stress affects a woman's heart differently than a man's. In one study out of Duke University School of Medicine where people were put in stressful situations, such as describing something that made them angry, the women were more likely than the men to show restricted blood flow to their hearts and increased blood clotting. These reactions are potentially life-threatening because they can lead to heart muscle damage and heart attacks.

While anything that kicks production of the stress hormone, cortisol, into high gear is bad for your health, constant conflict with people close to you can double, even triple, your risk of dying from any cause, compared to people with little friction in their lives.

The solution is to develop skills that will help you smooth out the rough spots in your relationships. Learn to manage anxiety, avoid squabbles, and reduce stress-inducing demands others make on you.

Don't worry, be happy. You need to take depression very seriously. It's a dangerous health condition with life-threatening consequences, hitting women and their hearts especially hard. In a three-year study of people suffering from depression, women younger than age 55 were twice as likely as others to suffer a heart attack or die from heart disease.

Other research suggests if you're older — past menopause — and suffer from depression, you're more likely to be overweight, carry that extra weight around your middle, and have high levels of inflammation. All three of these symptoms put you at higher risk of heart disease. Experts also wonder if hormones or chemical imbalances contribute to the link between these conditions.

Unfortunately, if you are depressed, you may find it difficult to make heart-healthy changes. What's the best do-it-yourself treatment for both your heart and your mental health? Exercise.

Take it off and keep it off. It's not just about you and your skinny jeans. It's about the number of fat cells in your body and what they are up to. Even if you're a good, "reasonable" weight, you've still got billions and billions of fat cells. They do important things like store energy, cushion fragile organs, help you absorb vitamins, and release compounds that activate your immune system. Too much fat, and your immune system goes into overdrive triggering inflammation everywhere — including your heart.

As a woman, even if you don't have any other risk factors, carrying too much weight puts you at a higher risk of heart disease. The Department of Medicine at Baylor College of Medicine says a modest amount of weight loss — just 7 percent — can be enough to swing the odds back in your favor. That's a mere 14 pounds for a 200-pound woman, and a perfect place to start.

Weight maintenance, however, may be your biggest hurdle. A recent study of 100 obese, postmenopausal women found those who lost weight, then regained most of it within a year were worse off than before. Their total cholesterol, LDL cholesterol, glucose, and insulin all climbed to levels higher than when they started.

Move even more. If you're a woman over age 30, being sedentary is probably the single greatest factor in developing heart disease. On the other hand, being even a little bit active could save your life, regardless of other risk factors. Just 30 minutes five days a week of moderate activity, like brisk walking, could cut your risk of heart disease by 14 percent.

Get 40 winks. Women need their sleep. And not just for beauty — for their hearts. Unfortunately, you have to get into a Goldilocks frame of mind and pin down the amount of sleep that is "just right," because both too little and too much are bad for you.

The University of Pennsylvania Perelman School of Medicine followed 86,000 peri- and postmenopausal women, ages 50 to 79. Whether the women got limited sleep, less than five hours a night, or a lot, more than 10 hours, they doubled their risk of heart disease during the 10-year study.

This is an emerging area of research. Experts realize there are many theories linking sleep and heart disease, but once more, the trouble may start with inflammation.

Your body views sleep deprivation as a time of stress. It reacts by ramping up your immune system, pumping out extra white blood cells, and triggering the inflammatory process.

In addition, during normal sleep times, your blood pressure drops to its lowest level. If you're sleep deprived, this never happens. When blood pressure stays elevated, your body, again, kicks into inflammation mode. If you already suffer from high blood pressure, missing even half a night's sleep can bump up your blood pressure the next day.

Can you ID a heart attack or stroke?

Sometimes you just have to ignore the tests and listen to your body. A study of 673 women with persistent chest pain found that even though an angiogram showed their arteries were not significantly blocked by plaque, in one year they experienced more than double the number of heart attacks and strokes as women without chest pain.

So if you've had discomfort anywhere above your waist, talk to your doctor. And learn the warning signs of a heart attack:

- pressure or squeezing in the center of your chest
- shortness of breath
- pain in one or both arms, your back, neck, or jaw
- nausea, dizziness, faintness, or a cold sweat

In addition, know these eight telltale symptoms that a stroke is underway or has occurred:

- sudden weakness or numbness in your face, arm, or leg, especially on one side of your body
- mental confusion or loss of memory
- vision loss or blurred vision
- slurred speech or inability to speak
- problems understanding other people
- an unexpected, severe headache
- unexplained dizziness, falls, or suddenly losing consciousness
- nausea and vomiting, especially when accompanied by any of these other symptoms

If you think you are having a heart attack or a stroke, it's vital you take prompt action by calling 911 immediately.

When leg pain signals heart trouble

Tell your doctor your chest hurts and you'll get his full attention. Say your legs hurt when you walk, and you may get the brushoff, "It's probably muscle aches or arthritis." This is a disturbing scenario, since you could be suffering from a life-threatening condition called peripheral artery disease or PAD.

Plaque isn't picky about where it causes problems, and if you have atherosclerosis, it's likely to block the arteries in your legs, restricting blood flow and oxygen. Your calves, thighs, or hips can cramp, become numb, or feel heavy, especially when walking or climbing stairs. Rest a while and the pain goes away, only to return when you walk again.

If you're concerned, ask your doctor to measure the blood pressure in your ankle, then compare it to an arm reading. This will show if your leg arteries are clogged. Left untreated, PAD puts you at higher risk of gangrene, amputation, heart attack, and stroke.

The first line of treatment for PAD is to stop smoking, since this is the greatest risk factor. A half-a-pack-a-day habit can increase your risk by 30 to 50 percent. While you may need medication to lower cholesterol, thin your blood, or reduce blood pressure, several safe and natural lifestyle changes could turn this condition around.

Redesign your diet. Take a hard look in your refrigerator, your pantry, and your lunchbox. Ditch anything that contributes to artery disease like saturated fat, sodium, and high-cholesterol foods. Choose foods high in fiber; antioxidant vitamins A, C, and E; folate; omega-3 fatty acids; and vitamin D — nutrients that are linked to fewer cases of PAD. In fact, the Mediterranean diet, rich in healthy fats like olive oil, could be a perfect solution. Researchers found it cut risk of PAD by 64 percent over a five-year period.

Take a stroll. For someone with PAD, a walking program may seem daunting at first, but clinical studies show it can improve the way your muscles pull oxygen from your blood and increase the number of blood vessels in your legs. Start slow, stopping to rest when you experience leg pain, then resume walking. Gradually increase how often you walk and for how long. In one study, people were able to walk farther and faster even a year after the trial ended. For safety, have a buddy close by whether you walk outdoors or on a treadmill.

Amazingly, working out your arms may be just as beneficial. A Minnesota study found that arm cycling improved general physical health, cardio fitness, and walking ability in people suffering from PAD. This could be a great addition to your workout routine that gets your heart rate up and boosts blood flow.

2 vaccines that could save your heart

Need another reason to get your vaccinations this year? Here are two.

- A flu shot could slash your risk of a heart attack, stroke, or heart failure within the next year — by a third if you have a history of heart disease and by as much as 50 percent if you've had a recent heart attack. Experts aren't completely sure how the vaccine protects you, but they think it may trigger your immune system to produce heart-defending proteins.
- Get the pneumonia vaccine and you protect your heart against tiny lesions caused by the *Streptococcus pneumoniae* bacteria. According to Carlos Orihuela, associate professor of microbiology and immunology at the University of Texas Health Science Center, a case of severe pneumonia could leave your heart permanently scarred and possibly explain the link between this dangerous infection and heart failure.

Cancel out your cancer risk

Smart ways to beat cancer: the lifestyle connection

Nothing strikes as much terror as a cancer diagnosis. And nothing inspires as much as personal stories of struggle and triumph over this deadly disease. Like Arthur, a 59-year-old diagnosed with aggressive prostate cancer who decided the worst thing he could do was sit around waiting for the next test.

So often it seems victory is a random combination of genetics, medical skill, and luck. But never discount the power you carry within. The power to make dramatic, life-saving health decisions. Arthur established his own eating and exercise program that made him feel he was doing everything he could to live a healthy life. Now he wakes up each morning with a sense of empowerment.

When you have cancer, you develop abnormal cells that divide and spread uncontrollably. Usually, they clump together, forming tumors that can invade and destroy tissues and organs around them. Sometimes these cells break off and travel to other parts of your body where they multiply to form new tumors. When this happens, your cancer has metastasized.

In order to beat cancer, the second leading cause of death in the United States, you must understand it runs much like an out-of-control car, cells growing and dividing as if the gas pedal is firmly stuck to the floor. Your job is to find the brake.

The World Cancer Report 2014 focused on four lifestyle behaviors that really rev the cancer engine — using tobacco, drinking alcohol, not exercising, and being obese. The first two are fairly straightforward. If you smoke or use any type of tobacco product, stop. And the researchers with the European Prospective Investigation Into Cancer and Nutrition study say your risk of cancer increases with every drink you take.

Here's the latest evidence on how two other healthy choices could save your life.

Lose weight. Experts believe that in just one year, there are at least 85,000 new cases of cancer in the U.S. due to obesity. One of the largest studies of weight and cancer risk found if you carry extra pounds, you have boosted your odds of developing 10 common cancers — uterine, gallbladder, kidney, liver, cervical, thyroid, leukemia, colon, ovarian, and breast.

Exactly how extra body fat affects the action of cancer cells is not completely understood, but the American Cancer Society suggests it may have something to do with:

- chronic low-level inflammation.
- proteins that influence how you use certain hormones.
- higher levels of hormones, like insulin and estrogen, that are linked to certain cancers.
- factors that control cell division, such as insulin-like growth factor-1 (IGF-1).

In addition, there's startling new research out of The University of Texas Health Science Center at Houston proposing a link between fat cells and tumor growth. They believe tumors attract special cells from fat tissue that help grow the blood supply these tumors need to survive.

The National Cancer Institute says if every adult reduced their BMI by just 1 percent, it would mean about 100,000 fewer new cases of cancer. To learn how to do this, read *Step 3: Lose the fat.*

Get active. Just being slim is not enough to ward off cancer. You need some level of fitness, as well. The American Cancer Society says everyone should get at least 150 minutes of moderate or 75 minutes of vigorous activity spread throughout the week. Experts are learning that being sedentary — or inactive — is a cancer danger all on its own. That means you must limit the amount of time you spend sitting, lying down, watching TV, or surfing the Internet.

Besides all the usual benefits — controlling weight; maintaining healthy bones, muscles, and joints; fighting high blood pressure; preventing diabetes; and just plain making you feel good — exercise can reduce your risk of the following cancers.

- Breast. Many types of breast cancer need estrogen to grow, and when you exercise, you reduce your body's levels of this hormone. Cardio workouts, which raise your heart rate, are especially good at breaking down cancer-promoting estrogen. For the same reason, exercise is also protective against other cancers related to estrogen, like ovarian and endometrial cancers.
- Colon. The less active you are, the slower your digestive system moves. And that means potential cancer-causing substances sit in your colon longer causing trouble. Experts think exercise could also protect you from colon cancer by reducing inflammation in your intestines, controlling insulin levels throughout your body, boosting your immune system, and pumping up your vitamin D when you exercise outside.
- Prostate. If you're a man, age 65 or older, and regularly exercise, you're 70 percent less likely to develop prostate cancer than men who don't work out. Being active lowers the amount of testosterone and other hormones in your blood that seem to stimulate the growth of prostate tumors. It also jump-starts your immune system and the natural antioxidant processes that help prevent this disease.

- Skin. There's an interesting relationship between exercising and skin cancer. Animal studies showed that when working out reduced the amount and thickness of fat layers in skin, there were fewer, smaller skin tumors.

Learn more about fun and easy ways to become active in *Step 4: Get up and move.*

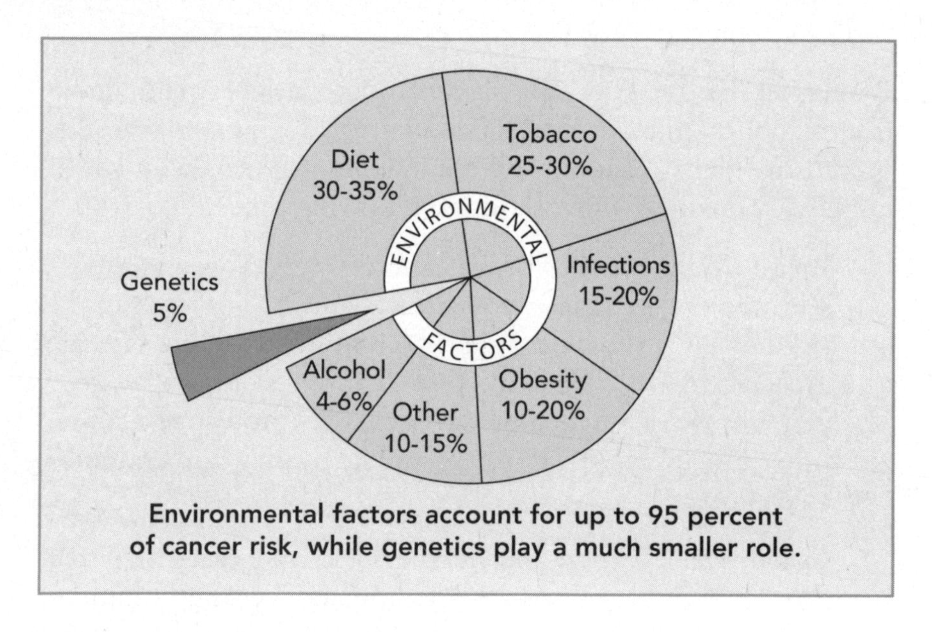

Environmental factors account for up to 95 percent of cancer risk, while genetics play a much smaller role.

Nutrition tips to lower your cancer risk

You can fight cancer and thrive by harnessing the awesome power of foods. All it takes is making some informed choices whether you're strolling through the supermarket, looking over a restaurant menu, or whipping up dinner in your own kitchen. Leading experts say for best health and cancer-fighting power eat whole foods and don't rely on dietary supplements. Here are some helpful guidelines.

Choose:

- whole grains when selecting breads, cereals, and pasta

- brown rice
- a variety of fruits, but especially those high in antioxidants like vitamin C and vitamin E
- an assortment of vegetables, including those containing specific phytochemicals known to fight cancer, like tomatoes and the cruciferous vegetables broccoli, cauliflower, and cabbage. Also pick vegetables high in antioxidants like vitamin C, vitamin E, and beta carotene.
- lean protein like chicken and fish
- garlic and onions
- vitamin-D rich foods like fortified milk and cereals

Avoid or limit:

- processed meats like bacon, sausage, lunch meats, and hot dogs, which contain salt, nitrites, and other compounds linked to cancer
- red meat high in saturated fat like beef, pork, and lamb
- alcohol to no more than two drinks a day for men and one drink a day for women — with one drink equaling 12 ounces of beer, 5 ounces of wine, or 1.5 ounces of hard liquor
- refined grains like white bread, since processing removes fiber and important nutrients
- sugar-sweetened beverages like sodas and sports drinks
- fruit or vegetable drinks that are not 100-percent juice
- white rice
- processed and sweetened snacks like candy and pastries
- salt and high-salt foods

Be sure to read *Step 2: Eat to Heal* for important nutrition information, as well as some specific news on foods that battle cancer.

An aspirin a day keeps cancer at bay

More than 40 years ago, researchers discovered when blood loses its ability to clot, cancer cells cannot easily spread, or metastasize. Decades later, aspirin, one of the most widely used anti-clotting medications, is still under review as a safe, effective way to lower your risk of cancer.

The most convincing evidence concerns colon cancer. It's long been known that aspirin protects your colon by preventing the formation of intestinal polyps, which can turn into cancer. The question has always been how. One theory is that it blocks your body from creating prostaglandins, chemicals important to these precancerous growths. New studies suggest aspirin also causes mutated intestinal stem cells to die. The theory is, take a daily aspirin and you'll not only reduce your risk of developing colon cancer, but improve your chances of surviving it.

Here's even more compelling evidence that aspirin is a serious cancer-fighter.

- Women who take a daily aspirin could reduce their risk of ovarian cancer by 20 percent, compared to those who use aspirin less than once a week.
- Yale researchers say they have evidence the longer someone takes low-dose aspirin, the smaller their chances of developing pancreatic cancer. In studies, a 10-year aspirin habit cut this risk in half.
- The famous Women's Health Initiative, involving close to 60,000 women ages 50 to 79, reports aspirin protected against melanoma, the deadliest form of skin cancer, possibly by controlling inflammation.
- Barrett's esophagus is a precancerous condition usually linked to ongoing acid reflux and affecting the tube that carries food from your mouth to your stomach. Some people with Barrett's are more likely than others to have this condition turn into

full-blown esophageal cancer. Aspirin may tip the odds in their favor by restricting cancer cell growth.

In addition, aspirin helps fight head, neck, throat, endometrial, and liver cancers.

A close look at all the current research leads experts to believe low-dose aspirin — anywhere from 75 to 325 milligrams daily — can give you some protection against various cancers if taken for at least five years. But because aspirin keeps your blood from clotting, it also raises your risk of dangerous bleeding and stroke. Ask your doctor if long-term aspirin therapy is right for you.

Embrace coffee's anti-cancer perks

Need another reason to love that cup of coffee? You'll live longer.

The National Institutes of Health – American Association of Retired Persons Diet and Health Study involving over 400,000 men and women, found those who fill it to the rim were less likely to die from heart disease, stroke, diabetes, respiratory disease, and infections than noncoffee drinkers. Now experts say that protection extends to cancer.

It might not be the caffeine. It may not even matter how you brew it. But in most cases, it does seem that more is better.

So go ahead and indulge your coffee passion and strike one against colon, endometrial, liver, oral, prostate, skin, and breast cancers.

Cancer screening sparks controversy

Will you automatically agree to a cancer screening your doctor suggests? Should you worry about overscreening? False positives? You may hear a different philosophy depending on who you talk to — your insurance company, a cancer survivor, a consumer advocate, a statistician, or even a medical researcher.

The National Cancer Institute identifies four different kinds of screening tests. They were designed to help find cancer in its earliest stages — when it's easier to treat and often before you have any symptoms.

- Physical exam. Your doctor will check your body for any signs of disease, such as lumps, tenderness, or skin changes.
- Laboratory tests. Samples of your blood, urine, tissue, or other substances are sent to a lab where they look for chemical or biological indicators of cancer.
- Imaging procedures. Detailed pictures of areas inside your body help doctors diagnose and plan treatment. Examples are X-rays, ultrasounds, magnetic resonance imaging (MRIs), and computed tomography (CT) scans.
- Genetic tests. Some cancers, like breast cancer, are often linked to specific gene mutations.

Unfortunately, the guidelines on cancer screenings have become convoluted due, in part, to evolving technology. Tests have become more sensitive, detecting tiny potential cancers that often disappear on their own or end up being harmless.

Here's information on screenings for three major types of cancer. Just remember, only you can decide what is right for you.

Colon cancer. Affecting the lower part of your digestive system, colon cancer usually begins as small clumps of noncancerous cells called adenomatous polyps. In time, some of these polyps can become cancerous. You rarely have symptoms from colon polyps, which makes screening that much more important.

The U.S. Preventive Services Task Force (USPSTF) is an independent panel of medical experts who review screenings, counseling services, and preventive medications to make recommendations to doctors and patients. They say every 50-year-old should be screened for colon cancer by having either a colonoscopy, sigmoidoscopy, or fecal occult blood test but only until age 75. If you are at average risk of developing colon cancer, tests like these can cut your risk of developing late-stage cancer by 70 percent.

Breast cancer. The American Cancer Society recommends that mammograms for women start at age 40 and continue every year as long as you are in good health. There is recent debate, however, based on 50 years of research, over whether mammograms might do more harm than good. The concerns include overdiagnosis; overtreatment of benign tumors including surgery, chemotherapy, and radiation; increased risk of harmful side effects of that treatment; and no reduction in the number of advanced breast cancer cases.

Here are the new, and somewhat controversial, guidelines from the USPSTF:

- No routine screening mammography from ages 40 to 49 unless called for by individual circumstances.
- A mammogram every two years between the ages of 50 and 74.
- No clear evidence to either support or oppose mammograms for women over 74 years old.

Mammograms save lives, although many experts admit the screening has shortcomings. Until something better comes along, women need to understand the limitations and possible consequences so they can make informed decisions.

Prostate cancer. PSA is the acronym for prostate-specific antigen. This enzyme enters the bloodstream when there's something amiss in the prostate gland. It was an important discovery back in 1970 because the antigen tips off doctors that tumors are recurring in men who have been treated for prostate cancer. But in 1994, the U.S. Food and Drug Administration (FDA) approved the PSA test to screen for previously undetected prostate cancer.

Doctors hastily embraced it as a simple, no-harm-done addition to the routine blood tests conducted during a man's annual physical examination.

Over the next two decades, the incidence of early-stage prostate cancer rose dramatically, while deaths from late-stage prostate disease took a dive. And, not surprisingly, nearly a million healthy men with elevated PSAs but no symptoms of disease were frightened into unnecessary radical surgery to have their prostates removed. This left the majority of them struggling with a lifetime of impotence and incontinence. As a result, the PSA test has become one of the hottest and most contentious medical controversies of modern times.

You may be surprised to learn the USPSTF recommends against PSA-based screening for men in generally good health, regardless of age. This recommendation, however, does not apply to men suspected of having prostate cancer.

Crucial questions you must ask your doctor

The National Institutes of Health and Consumer Reports recently examined the role cancer screening plays in today's health care. Their results may surprise you — too many people are getting tests they don't need, while too few are getting tests that could save their lives. Everyone should ask these six questions before undergoing any test.

1. What is my risk for cancer compared with the average person?
2. Does this test often give inaccurate results?
3. Can I choose a different test?
4. What should I do if the results are positive?
5. Are there any dangers or side effects?
6. What can I do to get ready for this test?

Also ask your doctor how much the test will cost, and how long it will take to get the results. All of this information will help you make the best choice for your health.

Step 7: Form new habits

Breaking bad: choose habits that heal

New Year's resolutions rarely work. In fact, researchers out of the University of Scranton report only about 8 percent of people are successful in achieving their resolution. Knowing what you want to do or even what you should do is not the same as actually doing it. In part, experts say, that's because your unconscious habits are mostly in charge of your day-to-day existence.

You're probably not even aware of how many tasks you perform and decisions you make on autopilot — everything from how you fix your morning coffee, to which items you buy at the supermarket, and even what expressions you use in your daily speech. One study found that more than 40 percent of everyday actions are habits — not actual decisions.

Here's how a habit is formed. The first time you sat in a car on your own, someone told you to buckle your seat belt. Over time, the trigger of getting into a car prompted your action of buckling up. With every repeated action, nervous system cells, called neurons, fired in a specific way. Over time, a pattern of behavior was literally worn into your brain. Now when there is a behavior trigger — getting into a car — the thinking part of your brain actually disengages and the habit — buckling your seat belt — takes over. The power of habit is so strong, you may even find that sitting in a car without a seat belt just feels wrong.

What does this mean to your health? Let's go back to that New Year's resolution. If you were like the majority of people making pledges on January 1, you vowed to lose weight. The problem is, at some point in your life you decided what you like to eat, how much, and how often. Pretty soon, these decisions became habits and you stopped making choices. Your brain, itself, changed, and your eating habits were born.

The downside to habits, of course, is that they can kick in even when you dislike the consequences. For instance, do you automatically head for the cookie jar after dinner? Do you always eat your salad with cheese and a creamy dressing? In order to realize your goal of losing weight, you will have to tackle bad eating habits like these.

Just how many habits affect your overall health? Hundreds. Maybe thousands. And they involve every aspect of your life — not only diet and weight, but also choices involving medical care, prescription drugs, supplements, your environment, and leisure time.

If you are trying to make smarter choices in your life, any bad habit can be a powerful stumbling block. As Charles Duhigg says in his book *The Power of Habit: Why We Do What We Do in Life and Business*, "Transforming a habit isn't necessarily easy or quick. It isn't always simple. But it is possible."

First, you must look at your world with new eyes, evaluating everything you do. Don't think about breaking a bad habit, which is an extremely difficult proposition involving its own set of mental processes. Instead, commit to replacing an old, unhealthy habit with a new, healthy one. This is important because experts say it is impossible to form a habit for not doing something. In other words, you want to create a new habit that will block an old one. Make it a small, manageable change, and choose a consistent time or place that will become your trigger. Be specific.

For instance, if your goal is to challenge your mind more, instead of saying, "I'm giving up watching TV," start small. Replace one hour of TV watching every morning with an hour spent working a crossword puzzle. Hook it onto a behavior trigger, like getting the morning paper or pouring a bowl of cereal. Soon, your breakfast routine will naturally include a healthy, brain-stimulating activity.

Here are some proven points you might not know about habits.

- Contrary to popular opinion, it does not take 21 days to form a new habit. It takes around 10 weeks — with daily repetition — for an action to become habit.
- You're much more likely to succeed in forming a new habit if you reward yourself immediately after the new action. That's because the prospect of a reward signals your brain to release dopamine, a feel-good chemical that also strengthens habits. For instance, if you hate going to the doctor, celebrate with lunch at your favorite restaurant after your appointment. Or just give yourself a mental pat on the back. Whatever works for you.
- Forgive yourself when you slip up. Studies show you'll bounce back and be more likely to establish that new habit if you don't punish yourself for failures.

Become more conscientious

Are you dependable and well-organized? What about prudent? Persistent? Maybe even just a little bit obsessive? Congratulations. You are more likely to live a long and healthy life.

Don't think of these stuffy, slightly boring-sounding traits as negative. They mean you are conscientious. According to results from an 80-year-long study, this tendency to do things well and thoroughly translates into health and longevity.

The now-famous Longevity Project, which began in 1921, followed over 1,500 children from the time they were 11 years old. Their personality traits were recorded throughout the years, and later researchers related these traits to health conditions and life span. They found:

- children who were dependable and thoughtful about the future lived the longest.

- as they grew to young adults, those who were thrifty, persistent, detail-oriented, and responsible lived the longest.

Having a conscientious personality also leads you into healthier situations and relationships. You're more likely to find your way to a happier marriage, better friendships, and healthier work situations.

There's nothing stopping you from nudging your personality or lifestyle in this direction. Here are some health-protecting habits conscientious people do naturally, or learn to do over time.

- wear a seat belt
- drink only in moderation
- don't abuse drugs
- follow doctors' orders
- generally avoid high-risk activities
- work hard
- follow a schedule
- don't smoke
- take medication as prescribed
- don't drive too fast
- get organized
- stay involved
- be prepared

Be a smarter patient

Do you take an active role in your own health? Part of that is knowing your family's medical history, keeping tabs on your blood pressure and cholesterol numbers, and realizing when you need a second opinion. It means you are making informed choices every step of the way. It also means preparing for your next medical appointment.

Know when you need a new doctor. Getting the best health care often starts with a good doctor-patient relationship. But remember, your doctor is working for you. Don't be intimidated by him or his staff. Their job is to help you stay well and healthy.

If they aren't doing that, fire them. Here are five warning signs you might need to change providers.

1. You are continually prescribed medications without any discussion of natural or lifestyle treatment options, including diet and exercise.
2. Your doctor does not seem up-to-date on new treatments.
3. You can never understand his medical explanations or instructions.
4. He always seems rushed.
5. He doesn't listen to you or value your input.

Learn how to talk to your doctor. You may think he doesn't listen to you, but could you be part of the problem? If you start your appointment with a long, rambling discussion of your aches and pains, the weather, your kids, and then your kidneys, don't be surprised if he seems to miss the point. But if you show up prepared, perhaps with written notes, you'll get his attention.

Most doctor's visits last 20 minutes or less, but you've got only about 20 seconds to present your most important point before the average doctor makes a mental diagnosis and interrupts your story.

Practice what you want to say before you go. Try it out in front of a family member, a friend, or even the mirror. And make sure to state your chief complaint early in your story, then follow it up with the facts in chronological order.

Never go to the hospital alone. Medical mistakes kill more people than car accidents or breast cancer. But you can protect yourself from hospital errors, prescription misunderstandings, confusing instructions, and a faulty memory by having someone with you to listen and take notes.

Don't have a friend or family member you can call on? Contact the patient advocate at your hospital. Their job is to resolve all concerns, make sure you get the care you need, and guarantee your voice is heard.

10 must-do health screenings

If part of being conscientious is planning ahead, you can check off that box by making the following appointments now. These vital health screenings are too important to brush aside, especially for women over age 65.

- Schedule an exam and cleaning with your dentist.
- Get your vision checked and ask about a glaucoma test.
- Plan a bone density test.
- Get a flu shot.
- Check if you need a tetanus booster.
- Go in for a shingles vaccination if you haven't already.
- See your primary care doctor for a physical.
- Ask if you are due for a mammogram or colonoscopy.
- Check your cholesterol levels and blood pressure numbers.
- Schedule a hearing test.

Practice good posture

Good posture does more than make you look good. It can make you feel good, too.

Boost your confidence. Sitting or standing in a straighter, more upright position is often called a power pose, and for good reason. When your head is up and your chest is out, you look and feel more self-assured. A study in the *European Journal of Social Psychology* found when people sat this way, they even described themselves differently — more positively — than people who sat slumped, in an uncertain posture.

Want to translate this into action? Practice a standing power pose in front of the mirror. Pull yourself as tall as possible, keeping your hands at your sides and your weight slightly forward, as if you're relaxed but ready for action. Or widen your stance and place your hands on your hips. Hold either of these poses for a couple of minutes and science shows you are actually increasing your testosterone levels, which, in turn, helps bump up your confidence.

Simply changing your body posture this way can give you a feeling of power and help you act more assertively.

Lift your mood. When you're looking and feeling confident and unafraid, it's easier to banish negativity. Try facing stress without slouching and you can change the way your body reacts. A New Zealand study found posture affected blood pressure and heart rate, making slumpers feel fearful, hostile, and nervous. Those sitting tall had a stronger pulse and a more positive mood.

Experts believe you can also apply this to soothing emotional pain. A dominant body position, where you take command of the space around you, could make a painful memory or emotional event less distressing.

Triumph over pain. Over 100 million Americans suffer from chronic pain. Whether it's a headache or a backache, your pain doesn't have to be crippling to be worthy of attention. And even though your instinct is to huddle in on the pain, fight it. A commanding posture — shoulders back, chest out, head up — helps you breathe deeply, gives you a sense of power and control over the pain, and can even affect hormones that will help you cope.

Physically, if you find your "neutral spine," the natural position where everything from your head and neck to your pelvis is in good alignment, you'll reduce strain on your back and relax tensed, aching muscles.

Live long and well. Britain's United Chiropractic Association believes poor posture is as bad for your health as obesity. In addition, studies show the more hunched you are:

- the more restricted your breathing.
- the more strain there is on your heart.
- the more help you'll need as you age to accomplish daily tasks like dressing and bathing.
- the less likely it is you will be able to live independently when you're older.

Increase your Rx IQ

The moment your doctor hands you a prescription is perhaps the most critical time to become an informed consumer. A few simple questions about a new medication could not only save you money and make you feel better, but could save your life.

Double-check the spelling. Do you know the difference between Flomax and Volmax? The first is a drug to relieve symptoms of an enlarged prostate. The second is for asthma. They sound alike. They have similar spellings.

But take the wrong one and you could end up in the hospital. Since 2000, the Food and Drug Administration (FDA) has received more than 95,000 reports of medication errors, many due to similar sounding names. The Institute for Safe Medication Practices recently updated their list of confused drug names, and came up with nearly 400 look-alike and sound-alike name pairs.

Protect yourself by asking your doctor to print the name and dosage of any new drug for you. Then check the label on your prescription at the pharmacy before leaving.

Understand the risks. Do you know the three medications responsible for the most drug-related emergency hospitalizations in seniors? They are:

- anticoagulants, like warfarin, and antiplatelets, like Plavix, which are both used to prevent blood clots and strokes in people with heart and blood vessel disease
- insulin, an injectable hormone used to treat diabetes
- oral hypoglycemics, a therapy for diabetes, used to stimulate cells in the pancreas to produce more insulin

These are valuable, often lifesaving drugs, so don't react rashly. Your job, as a patient, is to be sensible, thoughtful, and informed. If you're prescribed these or another drug, ask about side effects and interactions, and be absolutely certain you understand the dosage.

Request a generic alternative. If surveys accurately reflect what is happening across the country, doctors are likely to prescribe a brand name over a generic drug if you ask for it. This may seem like a puzzling scenario, but a recent questionnaire sent to close to 2,000 doctors — in internal medicine, family practice, pediatrics, cardiology, general surgery, psychiatry, and anesthesia — found that more than a third would honor this type of patient request. Consumer advocates are quick to point out that means more than half those surveyed would write a script for a generic, no matter what.

Working against generics is the flood of brand-name drug advertisements on television and in print. As a patient, you may be swayed by these direct-to-consumer ads. In fact, the FDA says these ads do a good job of raising awareness of conditions and possible treatments. Just realize the risks and benefits may not be equally communicated.

The bottom line is you should ask either your doctor or your pharmacist if there is a generic equivalent of any medicine you take, and if it would be a good alternative for you.

Steer clear of germs

Unless you live in a plastic bubble, you can't completely avoid the millions of tiny, infection-causing microbes in the world around you. But there are lots of little things you can do to help protect yourself and others from spreading these germs.

Sneeze into your elbow. Which is worse — watching someone cough or sneeze without covering their face, or watching them use their hand as a shield? Of course, neither strategy is hygienically correct. But after learning the results of a new study published in the *Journal of Fluid Mechanics*, you may never go out during flu season again.

Massachusetts Institute of Technology researchers explain there is an invisible gas cloud you expel with every cough or sneeze that propels droplets of mucus 200 times further than previously thought and allows them to stay airborne long enough to enter ventilation units.

If you're sick and must mingle, cover your mouth and nose with your shoulder or your elbow when you cough or sneeze. If you're healthy, stay at least 8 feet from the hacker.

Greet with a fist bump. It's not just for the young and hip. This gentle knocking of knuckles may be the healthiest new way to say hello. The traditional handshake, especially long, firm grips like your father taught you, means fingertips and palms meet. Eventually, your hand touches your eyes or mouth, more people, and other surfaces, spreading 10 times more bacteria than the quick tap of a closed fist.

Washing your hands frequently and thoroughly is the best way to keep from spreading germs, but since even hospital workers do it properly only 40 percent of the time, fist-bumping is a simple, hygienic alternative.

Clean your cellphone. They go with you to the gym, the dinner table, the restroom, and even your bed. They nestle up close and personal to your cheek, eyes, mouth, and ears. So what's wrong with this picture? According to one report, cellphones carry 10 times more bacteria than most toilet seats.

The worst news is many cellphone manufacturers explicitly forbid you to clean them with liquid or aerosol cleaners. That's unfortunate because an independent lab found that plain, old rubbing alcohol can clean nearly 100 percent of the bacteria from your electronic device.

While microfiber cloths will remove oil and dirt, they can't rub off all bacteria. Still, you can find sanitizing wipes made for mobile devices. Use them at least once a week. Another alternative is to buy a product that uses UV-C light to zap bacteria in four minutes.

Buy your own yoga mat. Don't stop doing yoga. It's healthy in so many ways. But for less than $10, you can amp up its health factor by owning your own yoga mat. Shared mats are literally a breeding ground for bacteria. Think about it. They are usually stored in a warm, humid environment, their surfaces are full of tiny crevices, they are laid out on a floor where people walk barefoot, and then multiple exercisers — including you — step, lay, sweat, and roll around on them.

It's this direct skin contact that is so worrisome. The list of possible infections you could pick up read like a Who's Who of bacteria — herpes, plantar warts, MRSA, jock itch, toenail fungus, athlete's foot, and, of course, your basic cold and flu viruses.

Experts also advise you to follow what they call yoga hygiene:

- Clean the mat before and after you use it with a disinfecting spray or wipe. If that's not possible, cover it with a clean towel.
- Bandage any cuts or scrapes.
- Buy and use hand and foot mitts.

Take a probiotic

Bacteria have gotten a bad rap. You probably think of them as germs. And, in many cases, you would be right. But bacteria that live and thrive inside your body are so much more.

Your digestive system, especially, is home to an abundance of bacteria that help it work properly. These are sometimes called gut flora or intestinal microbiota. They help you digest, absorb, synthesize, and metabolize all kinds of nutrients and other substances. When you don't have enough good bacteria here you can often feel it, in the form of constipation, gas, diarrhea, or various infections.

But scientists are continuing to explore other areas of the body containing good bacteria and just how these microorganisms, known collectively as your microbiome, impact your health, including:

- sinusitis
- high cholesterol
- rheumatoid arthritis
- brain function
- allergies
- high blood pressure
- obesity

You can buy probiotics, which are live microorganisms similar to the ones you have naturally in your body. They come as capsules, tablets, or powders, and in certain foods, like yogurt. You would want to take probiotics for several reasons:

- to generally boost your immune system
- to replace the good bacteria killed off by disease, stress, poor diet, or a round of antibiotics
- to treat or prevent certain conditions or infections

When choosing a probiotic, select one with the type of bacteria shown to work for your complaint. Next, make sure you're getting enough live cells in every dose. Products can range from 100 million cells to 900 billion per dose. You'll have to do your homework here to determine what you need. And finally, remember there are some situations where taking probiotics is not a healthy decision, so talk to your doctor first.

Check expiration dates

The eternal dilemma — should you toss that bottle, can, or package that's been in the drawer for who knows how long? You'd like to trust the expiration date, but these can be alarmingly inaccurate, more like guidelines, really. Understanding date stamps can sometimes mean the difference between sickness and health.

Medications. The Food and Drug Administration (FDA) requires manufacturers to put an expiration date on all prescription and over-the-counter drugs. Generally, it means the medicine is guaranteed to be fully effective up to that date. On the other hand, an expired medicine may work just fine, and it's unlikely to hurt you.

What you'll want to do is evaluate the seriousness of your condition. If your life depends on a medication, make sure it is current and operating at full strength. Otherwise, give it a close inspection and use some common sense. Toss liquids or pills that smell bad, capsules that are cracked, and ointments that are hardened.

So what about those old drugs? Don't just dump them in your trash or flush them down the toilet. Dispose of them properly at your local pharmacy or through a collection program, like the National Prescription Drug Take-Back Day sponsored by the U.S. Drug Enforcement Administration.

Packaged foods. Except for infant formula, there are no federal regulations saying food products have to be date stamped. But many states do have dating requirements.

The United States Department of Agriculture (USDA) lists four types of food product dating:

- Sell-By. This tells the store how long to display the product for sale. Try to buy the product before this date expires.
- Best if Used By. For the best flavor or quality, use a product before this date.
- Use-By. The manufacturer recommends you eat the food before this date for peak quality.
- Closed or coded dates. These are packing numbers used by the manufacturer.

It can be a confusing exercise decoding the different recommendations, but *Consumer Reports* suggests you follow sell-by and use-by dates at least on dairy and meat products. Otherwise, it's a personal choice, often requiring a little background knowledge. For instance, olive oil does not get better with age. Over time, the heart-healthy compounds break down. So if a bottle is date-stamped, especially with a harvest date, let that guide you.

Cosmetics. If unopened, most body products and makeup are good for about two to three years after you buy them. One exception is sunscreen, which has an expiration date on the package you should always abide by. The safe lifespan of opened products is surprisingly small. Mascara may be the trickiest, with experts suggesting you toss it after just three months.

The trouble begins as soon as that bath oil, lipstick, cream, or lotion is exposed to the air. Germs hovering over your sink or floating in that public restroom settle in and start to multiply. The longer and more often the container is open, the worse the problem.

Then there are the germs you add to the mix. You naturally have bacteria on your skin, lips, and eyes. If you're sick, that makes it even worse. And don't even consider sharing with another person. To minimize all this contamination, replace sponges weekly, wash brushes and other applicators every month, buy pump dispensers when possible, and seal all jars and bottles tightly after each use.

Say no to processed foods

"If it came from a plant, eat it; if it was made in a plant, don't." So says Michael Pollan, author of *The Omnivore's Dilemma*.

That's a lovely sentiment, but perhaps not so practical. Most items you buy in your supermarket, technically, come from a processing plant. They've been handled, washed, cut, and packaged — at the very least. But you'll learn there are degrees of processing. Hot dogs are processed, but then so is whole-wheat bread or a bag of spinach.

Avoid the worst offenders. In the best sense, processed foods are easy ways to get safe, complete nutrition. They are convenient time-savers that can have a long shelf life. In the worst sense, they are low in nutrients and high in calories; salt; sugar; refined flour; artificial flavorings, colorings, and sweeteners; and preservatives, like the nitrates in cured meats.

The following is not a scientific list. In fact, ask 10 different nutritionists and you'd probably get 10 very different lists. But these represent the type of processed foods you should avoid:

- soda
- hot dogs
- potato chips
- french fries
- snack cakes
- white bread
- candy bars
- cheese dips

What do they all have in common? They are heavily processed. Your first step toward better nutrition is to become smart on the levels of processing. The Academy of Nutrition and Dietetics explains them this way:

- Minimally processed foods, like cut vegetables and roasted nuts, are simply pre-prepped for convenience.

- Moderately processed foods, like canned tuna and most canned and frozen fruits and vegetables, make the most of their nutritional benefits while extending their shelf life.
- More heavily processed foods have ingredients added for flavor and texture, like sweeteners, spices, and oils, as well as colors and preservatives. Examples are jarred pasta sauce, salad dressing, yogurt, and ready-to-eat foods, like crackers, granola, and deli meat.
- The most heavily processed foods include frozen pizza and microwaveable dinners, as well as unhealthy snack foods like those in the list.

Strive for healthy habits. Here are some smart and easy ways to avoid processed foods.

- Shop only the perimeter of your grocery store, where you're more likely to find whole foods like meat, dairy, and produce.
- Make friends with your produce manager. Ask about seasonal fruits and vegetables, and the best way to select and prepare them. Learn about new or unusual produce you might not normally buy.
- Read ingredient lists and remember they are in descending order. The first few ingredients are those you'll be getting the most of.
- Learn how to decipher nutrition labels. This way you can eliminate items with too much salt, sugar, fat, and other unhealthy ingredients. See the chapter *Food smarts: heroes to zeroes* for more information.
- Shop at a farmer's market.
- Limit boxed and canned food items. Even those that seem harmless, like instant noodles, can be crammed with sodium and unhealthy saturated fat.

- Restrict your beverages to water, 100-percent juices, coffee, tea, and milk.
- Ban most fast food and all deep-fried foods.
- Make your own lunches.
- Whip up your own smoothies. Commercial ones have lots of added sugar. By blending your own, you control the calories.

Protect yourself from the sun

Skin cancer is a highly preventable disease, yet one out of every five people in the United States will develop it during their lifetime. It most often occurs in basal and squamous cells in the outer layer of your skin, usually on sun-exposed areas like your face, ears, neck, lips, and the backs of your hands. If detected early enough, this type of skin cancer is easily treated, but you can avoid it altogether by following these simple steps.

Slather on sunscreen. It's not true the majority of dangerous skin damage is done before the age of 18, as many people believe. In fact, as you age, your cells aren't as capable of repairing damage caused by sun exposure and the cancer-fighting ability of your immune system naturally weakens. That means it's never too late to use sunscreen. Just remember these tips.

- Use enough. The American Cancer Society says if you're average size, you should apply about 1 ounce of sunscreen, the amount it would take to fill a shot glass, on your arms, legs, neck, and face.
- Apply it 15 to 30 minutes before going out in the sun.
- Reapply at least every two hours, and more often if you sweat or swim.

- Wearing sunscreen doesn't give you a free pass to spend as much time as you like in the sun. Limit exposure especially during the middle of the day.

Perform a self-exam. The Skin Cancer Foundation recommends you give yourself a head-to-toe checkup every month, looking for new or changing moles or anything unusual that might be cancerous or precancerous. Be thorough, using a mirror to examine those hard-to-reach areas. In addition, go to a dermatologist every year for a checkup, more often if you find something suspicious.

Nix indoor tanning. That year-round bronzed look can be deadly. It increases your risk of melanoma, the deadliest form of skin cancer, even if you never experience a sunburn.

Limit eye damage. The most delicate skin on your body is around your eyes, with up to 10 percent of all skin cancers found on the eyelid. But you must also protect the eye, itself, from the sun's harmful rays. They can cause cancers within your eye, as well as vision-stealing cataracts and the incurable eye disease, macular degeneration.

Buy sunglasses that block 99 to 100 percent of ultraviolet A (UVA) and ultraviolet B (UVB) rays. Choose large lenses that offer protection to the sides of your eyes and fit close to your face.

Manicure safely. Some nail salons use ultraviolet light to speed-dry gel nail polish, exposing your hands to the same harmful radiation emitted by tanning beds. Researchers admit the lamps they tested varied in wattage, so they calculated that an average of 11 sessions under the light would raise cancer risk. In actuality, it could take anywhere from eight to 208 minutes to deliver a damaging dose of radiation.

Ask your salon what type of lamp they use, and if you decide to proceed with a gel manicure, put sunscreen on your hands or wear UV-protective gloves that cover all but your fingertips.

Try some nutritional defense. Bulk up your diet with smart menu choices and high-powered nutrients to help make your skin even more resistant to skin cancer.

- Selenium. This trace mineral acts as an antioxidant to neutralize free radicals. It may also rev up immune cells to help keep tumors from growing. Good sources of selenium include Brazil nuts, canned light tuna, cod, and light meat turkey.
- Carotenoids. These naturally occurring pigments give red, yellow, or orange color to foods like tomatoes, carrots, and corn. When too much sun exposure produces dangerous free radicals in your skin, carotenoid antioxidants can counteract them on the spot.
- Resveratrol. This powerful compound, found in grapes, peanuts, wine, and grape juice, helps stop tumors from forming.
- Omega-3 fatty acids. Researchers suspect that fish rich in omega-3s protect your skin against damage from inflammation, especially the kind caused by the sun. Enjoy oily fish like salmon, herring, sardines, or trout every week.
- Green or black tea. The polyphenols in green tea, especially, may help your skin wield an arsenal of weapons against the sun damage that triggers skin cancer. A study from Dartmouth Medical School in New Hampshire found that people who drank two or more cups of green or black tea a day for at least a month cut their risk of two types of skin cancer — squamous cell carcinoma and basal cell carcinoma — by 20 to 30 percent.

Avoid these 10 environmental toxins

Compounds found in everyday consumer products can be hazardous to your health. The Centers for Disease Control and

Prevention (CDC) currently measures more than 300 environmental chemicals to see how much people are exposed to through air, water, food, soil, dust, or consumer products. This is called biomonitoring.

The list of potential hazards is full of unpronounceable words, like N,N-Diethyl-meta-toluamide, which you may know as DEET, an insect repellant first marketed in 1957 that can cause skin and neurological problems.

If you were to learn about each chemical, how it impacts human health, and where it can be found, you might book a seat on the first spaceship off the planet.

But don't give up hope. Despite the increasing number of chemicals introduced by manufacturers every year, governments are working to regulate their safety. Along with the CDC, the National Toxicology Program, part of the U.S. Department of Health and Human Services; the Environmental Protection Agency (EPA); the Food and Drug Administration (FDA); and other organizations study, test, and promote safe levels of these environmental toxins.

Focus on the things you can control right now. Switch to nontoxic and natural alternatives for products you use on your body and in and around your home.

Bisphenol A (BPA). BPA is used in polycarbonate plastics, epoxy resins, and in certain thermal paper products, including some cash register and ATM receipts. To reduce your exposure to BPA, the National Toxicology Program offers these tips:

- Avoid plastic containers with the #7 or the letters "PC" on the bottom.
- Stop microwaving food in polycarbonate plastic containers. Over time, the chemical can break down from the high temperatures.

- Wash polycarbonate plastic containers by hand. Avoid your dishwasher's harsh detergents.
- Eat fresh or frozen foods and rely less on canned foods.
- Choose glass, porcelain, or stainless steel containers, especially for hot food and liquids.
- Buy baby bottles and toys labeled BPA free.

Atrazine. This agricultural pesticide is widely used in the U.S. It's sometimes used on residential lawns, especially in Florida and the Southeast. Buy a water filter certified to remove atrazine from your drinking water, and choose organic fruits and vegetables.

Phthalates. These chemicals, often called plasticizers, are used to make plastics more flexible and harder to break. Avoid plastic food containers, children's toys, and plastic wrap made from PVC, which has the recycling label #3. Some soap, shampoo, hair spray, and nail polish also contain phthalates. Always read labels and avoid products that list added "fragrance." This general term sometimes means hidden phthalates.

Flame retardants. Added to furniture, clothing, building materials, and other products, these chemicals reduce the likelihood of fire. Ask before buying furniture if it contains flame retardant chemicals. Use a vacuum with a HEPA filter to cut down on toxic house dust. Take care when replacing old carpet since the padding underneath may contain toxins.

Arsenic. This highly poisonous element can cause bladder, lung, and skin cancer, and it may also cause kidney and liver cancer. It harms the central and peripheral nervous systems, as well as heart and blood vessels, and causes serious skin problems. It contaminates drinking water either from natural deposits in the earth or from industrial and agricultural pollution. Use a water filter that lowers arsenic levels.

Mercury. Methylmercury builds up in the tissues of fish, with larger and older fish usually having the highest levels. To limit your exposure, choose wild salmon and farmed trout.

Perfluorooctanoic acid (PFOA). This example of a perfluorochemical (PFC) is used on nonstick pans, as well as in stain and water-resistant coatings on clothing, furniture, and carpets.

Organophosphate pesticides. These pesticides affect the nervous system by disrupting the enzyme that regulates the neurotransmitter acetylcholine. Because some of these pesticides are very poisonous, avoid them by choosing organic produce.

Glycol ethers. You can be exposed to these through cleaning products, liquid soaps, and cosmetics. Avoid ingredients such as 2-butoxyethanol (EGBE), methoxydiglycol (DEGME), 2-methoxyethanol, and 2-ethoxyethanol.

Parabens. These chemicals are widely used as preservatives in cosmetics and personal care products, and as antimicrobials to prevent food spoilage. According to the European Commission's Scientific Committee on Consumer Products, some parabens can disrupt your endocrine system and cause reproductive and developmental disorders. Avoid these ingredients — methylparaben, propylparaben, butylparaben, or benzylparaben.

Engage your brain

Think of your brain as a muscle. Just like any other muscle in your body, you must follow the old adage of "use it or lose it." Give your brain its own trip to the gym and you could delay or slow the progress of Alzheimer's disease and other forms of dementia.

Years ago, experts thought each person was born with all the brain cells they would ever have. Then, not only did they learn you could form new cells throughout your life, but you could also change and rewire your brain based on knowledge and experience. So just as someone with little muscle tone in their arms and legs can exercise their way to a stronger and more fit body, you can work out your brain and enjoy sharper thinking.

Learn something new. Just 15 minutes a day learning something unfamiliar means your brain is building new cells and communication pathways. Challenge yourself with different activities, both physical and mental, and your brain responds by changing and growing, becoming better, faster, and leaner.

While doing harder crossword puzzles or tackling more complicated recipes in the kitchen will stretch your current abilities, challenging yourself with something unrelated is even better at building brainpower. For big benefits, have a go at something completely different from your existing strengths.

Have fun with games and puzzles. Roll your lucky dice, deal a winning hand, or count out those points — however you play, you can be sure you're coming in first when it comes to brainpower. Games aren't just for kids anymore. While you're sharpening your pencil, you'll be sharpening your thinking skills and slashing your risk of dementia.

Read. Of course, you read something every day. But amp it up and you'll make a deposit into your oh-so-important cognitive reserves. Choose material that makes you think or teaches you something new. Join a book club or reading group so you're forced to analyze and discuss what you've read. Look up unfamiliar words in the dictionary and mull over new ideas. Try an author or genre outside your comfort zone to add an element of change to the activity. All this builds vocabulary, memory, reading efficiency, and knowledge and can cut your risk of dementia.

Practice Neurobics. Is there a rebel hidden inside of you? Ever dream of throwing tradition to the wind and doing things in a completely new and challenging way? Here's your chance, and you'll be giving your brain a workout at the same time.

That's the concept behind Neurobics, a term coined by Lawrence Katz, Professor of Neurobiology at Duke University Medical Center, and Manning Rubin, a writer in the communications and advertising business. Neurobics describes exercises designed to increase your brain's ability to stay fit, learn, and remember.

Katz and Rubin claim that everyday life is the Neurobic brain gym. That means you can engage in Neurobic exercises anywhere and at anytime. Here are some examples.

- Brush your teeth with your left hand if you are right-handed.
- Get dressed with your eyes closed.
- Completely rearrange your office.
- Select the correct change from your coin purse without looking.
- Listen to a completely new genre of music.
- Drive somewhere familiar using a totally new route.

Socialize

You could live up to 22 percent longer just by having more friends. Socializing helps extend your life, fight depression, and ward off dementia.

In an Australian study, older people with the largest network of good friends were more likely to survive during the 10-year follow-up period. In fact, those with the most friends were 22 percent less likely to die than those with the least.

Researchers suspect friends may encourage older people to take better care of themselves. They may also help you get through tough times, boosting your mood and self-esteem. So make more friends, and make the most of your life.

Choose happy friends. A University of California San Diego study found that happiness is contagious. People surrounded by many happy people are more likely to become happy. If a friend who lives within a mile of you becomes happy, your odds of becoming happy increase by 25 percent. Researchers found similar effects for spouses, siblings who lived within a mile, and next-door neighbors.

Keep it small. You may not need a large circle of friends. Maintaining relationships with small groups of close friends or family members can also keep your mind sharp.

Talk it out. A University of Michigan study found that having a 10-minute conversation was just as effective as doing an intellectual activity in terms of boosting memory and mental performance. That means just visiting a neighbor or friend can be as helpful in keeping your brain sharp as doing a daily crossword puzzle. So can playing bridge, which combines mental activity with social interaction. On the other hand, remember, your connections don't always have to be face to face. You can keep in touch by phone, email, or letters.

Look for a little love. Romantic relationships also matter. An interesting recent study suggests that people who are unmarried or living alone during midlife may have an increased risk of developing Alzheimer's disease. Those who were married or lived with a significant other during midlfe had a 50 percent lower risk of developing dementia later in life.

Stay independent

Your quest for independence began the moment your parents let go of the handlebars. You moved further along the path when they waved goodbye at the bus stop, and never faltered until they handed over the car keys. You've probably spent your life cultivating that independence — and, perhaps, teaching it to others.

Don't let muscle weakness or aching joints rob you of this hard-won freedom. Make sure you stay strong and active in the coming years. One way is to improve your balance and reduce your risk of falling. The Centers for Disease Control and Prevention (CDC) reports that falls are the leading cause of injuries in older adults. Up to 30 percent of these injuries make it difficult, if not impossible, for people to get around and continue living independently.

You don't need special equipment or long, involved training. Just add strength and balance movements into your everyday activities.

- Squat instead of bending over to pick up your newspaper.
- Stand on one leg while making breakfast, ironing, or talking on the phone.
- Try walking sideways from room to room.
- Sit down in a chair without using your hands.

It may sound strange, but people who moved like this throughout the day had 31 percent fewer falls over a year compared to groups who exercised a few times a week, reported a study in the *British Medical Journal.* The movements were part of a program called Lifestyle Integrated Functional Exercise (LiFE).

The point of the LiFE approach is to become stronger and more stable by continuously challenging yourself to shift your weight, step over objects, turn and change direction, and use less physical support.

Here's another great balance-boosting exercise that may decrease your risk of falls and help keep your joints flexible. Walk in a circle or oval around your living room or yard for 10 to 15 minutes. Start with a large circle, and keep making it smaller so the curve becomes tighter. That will increase your challenge to stay balanced.

Practice good hygiene

Treat your body with loving care. Become more aware of what you can do to stay fit and healthy. A good first step is basic cleanliness, which has far-reaching health consequences.

Take care of your mouth. This means more than just a beautiful smile. It means a lower risk of tooth decay and gum disease, or periodontitis. And keeping bacteria from setting up shop in your mouth is more important than you may think. Chronic gum disease creates inflammation and is linked to:

- Alzheimer's disease
- pancreatic cancer
- heart disease, heart attack, and stroke
- knee osteoarthritis and rheumatoid arthritis
- respiratory diseases

So what is your plan of attack? Brush and floss twice a day, drink lots of water, and visit your dentist for regular exams and cleanings.

Wash your hands. The Centers for Disease Control and Prevention calls it a "do-it-yourself vaccine." When you wash your hands correctly, you remove germs you might otherwise transfer to your eyes, nose, and mouth, or pass on to food, surfaces, and other people. Scrub for a good 20 seconds — long enough to hum the "Happy Birthday" song twice.

Don't neglect your feet. Good foot care is not just for people with diabetes. Your feet support you, take you where you want to go, and allow you to exercise and have fun. Just because they exist way down at the end of your legs doesn't mean you should forget about them. Not only do you need to keep them clean and dry, the Institute for Preventive Foot Health says well-fitting shoes and socks, proper toenail care, and daily inspections are vitally important.

A

D

E

F

G

H

I

N

O

P

Q

R

S

T

U

V